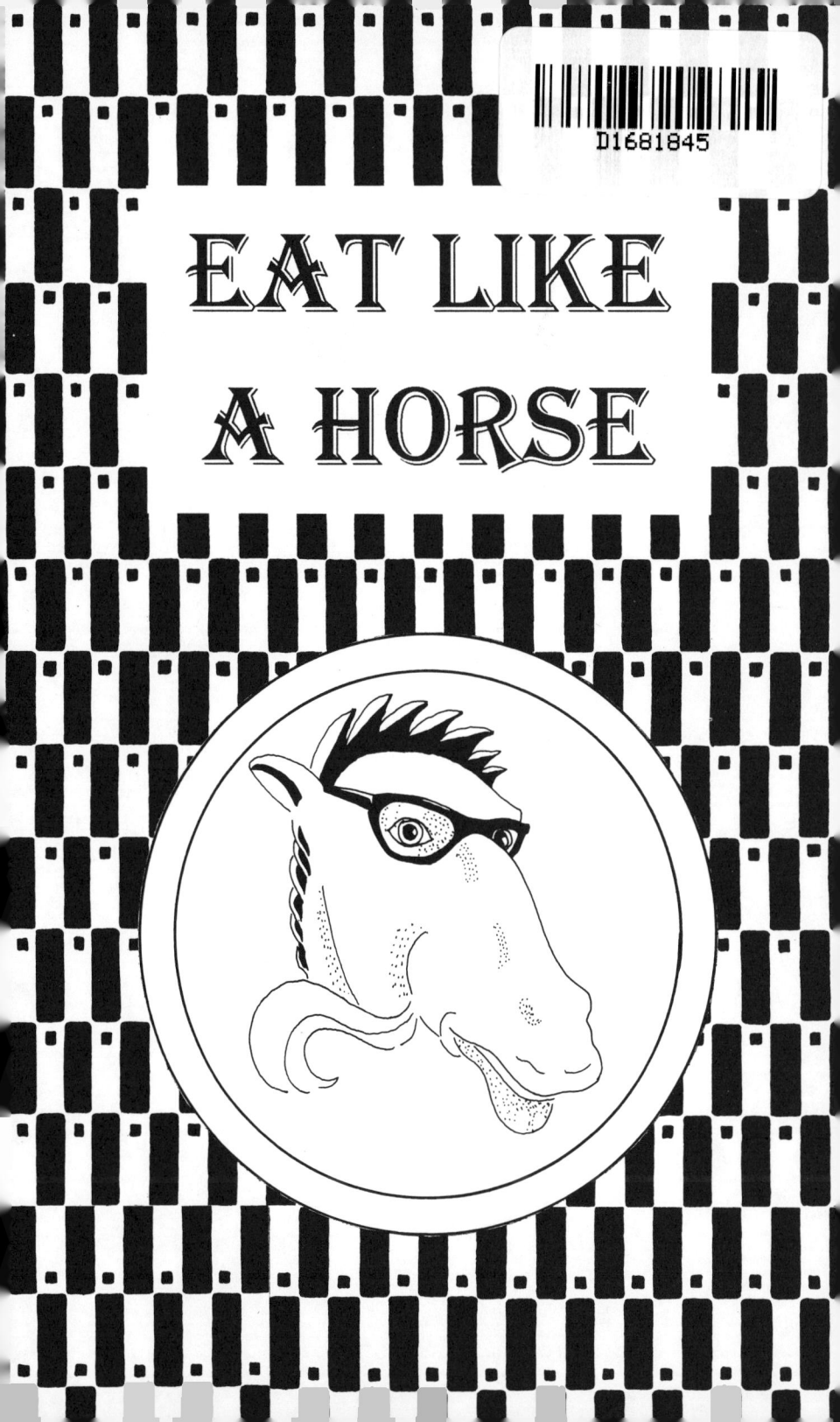

EAT LIKE A HORSE

EAT LIKE A HORSE AND LOSE WEIGHT

By

Barbara Richter

Illustrations by G.V. Pickup

AIRPLANE BOOKS

The author and publishers wish to remind you that it is sound practice to consult your physician before beginning any new dietary program.

Fat gram content of recipes: Nutritive Value of Foods, USDA, revised June, 1991; food packaging labels; and private sources.

All rights reserved. No part of this book may be reproduced or transmitted in any form or by any means, electronic or mechanical, including photocopying, recording, or by any information storage and retrieval system, without permission in writing from the author.

Text Copyright © 1994 Barbara Richter

Illustrations Copyright © 1994 G.V. Pickup

Published by Airplane Books
P.O. Box 111
Glenview, IL 60025

Publisher's Cataloging in Publication

Richter, Barbara F.
    Eat like a horse and lose weight / by Barbara Richter ; illustrations by G.V. Pickup.
    p. cm.
    Includes index.
    Preassigned LCCN: 94-077969
    ISBN 0-9641715-3-8

1. Low-fat diet--Recipes. 2. Cookery. I. Pickup, G.V., ill. II. Title.
RM237.7.R53 1994   641.5'638
                                    QBI94-1757

Printed in the United States of America

First Edition: October 1994

10 9 8 7 6 5 4 3 2 1

Dedicated to J. H.

Eat Like a Horse would not have been possible without the boundless efforts of very dedicated people. Most particularly and to whom we are very grateful is Jill Houk for her technical expertise and enthusiasm. Terry Nemeth for unfailingly steering us in the right direction. And we are very appreciative of our testers and tasters who ate like a horse and didn't gain weight in the line of duty; Ted Shell, Librada Perez, Mary Jo Ghiselli, Joy Nieda, Pat Mead, and Rita DiVito.

TABLE OF CONTENTS

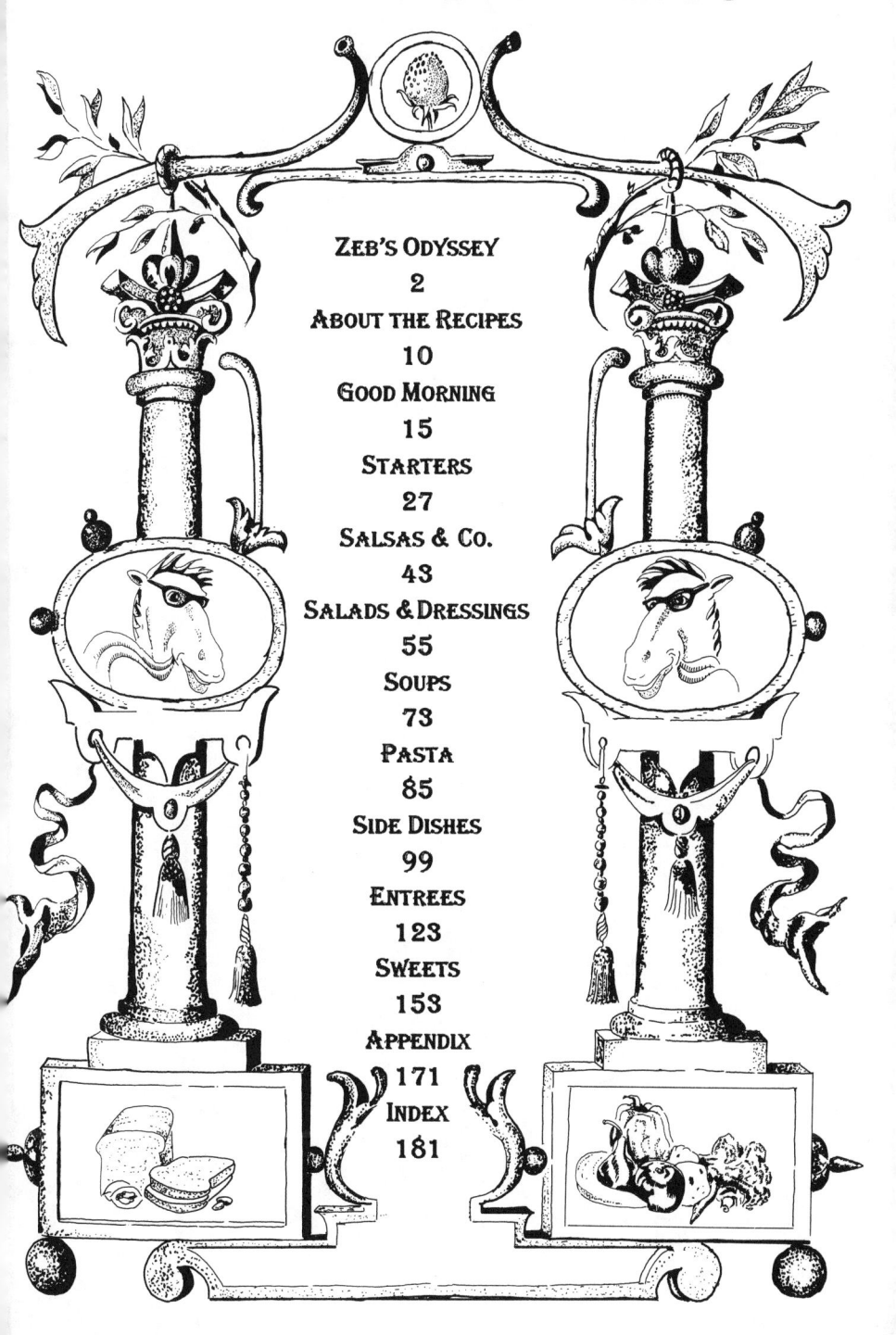

Zeb's Odyssey
2
About the Recipes
10
Good Morning
15
Starters
27
Salsas & Co.
43
Salads & Dressings
55
Soups
73
Pasta
85
Side Dishes
99
Entrees
123
Sweets
153
Appendix
171
Index
181

Zeb's Odyssey

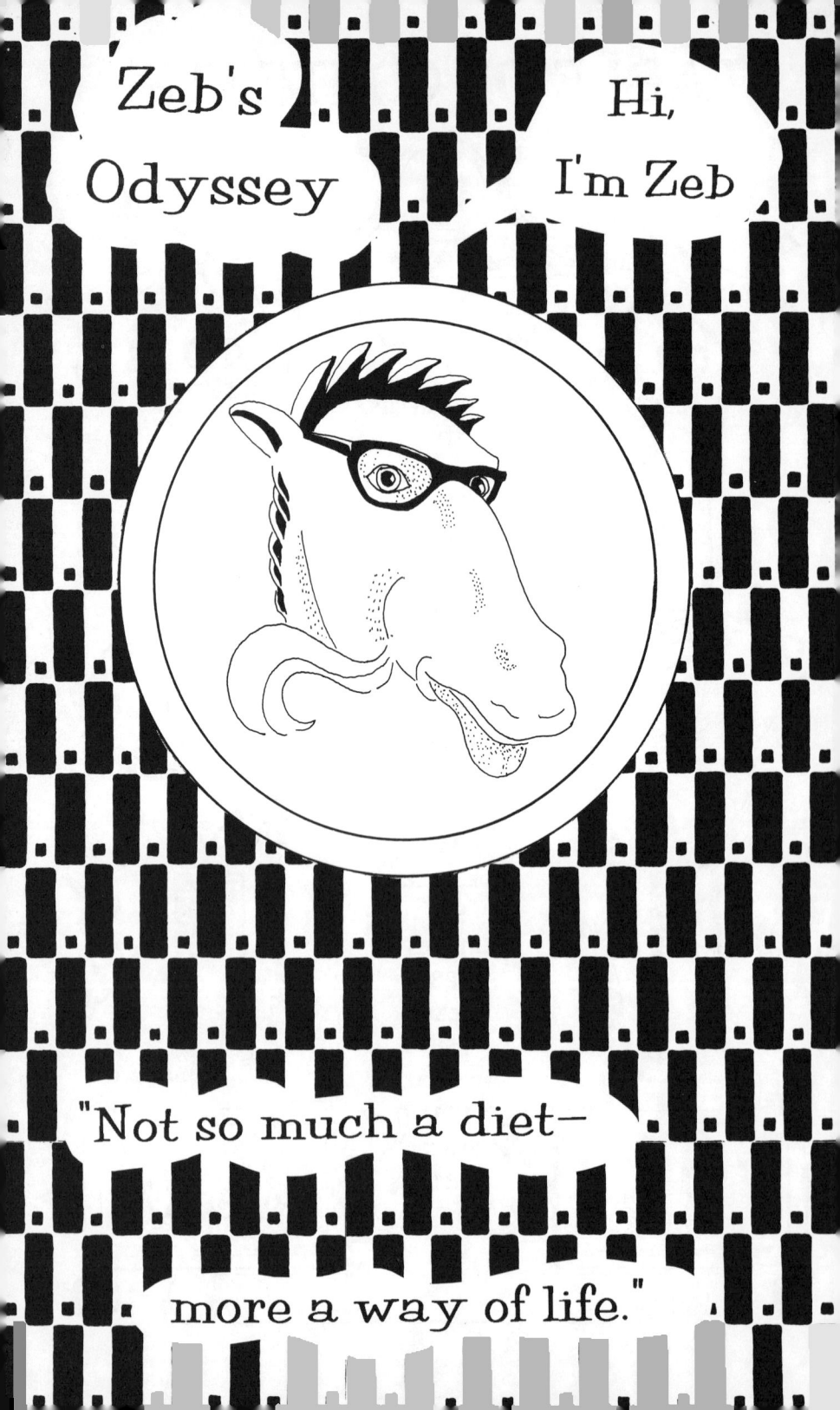

Hi, I'm Zeb

"Not so much a diet— more a way of life."

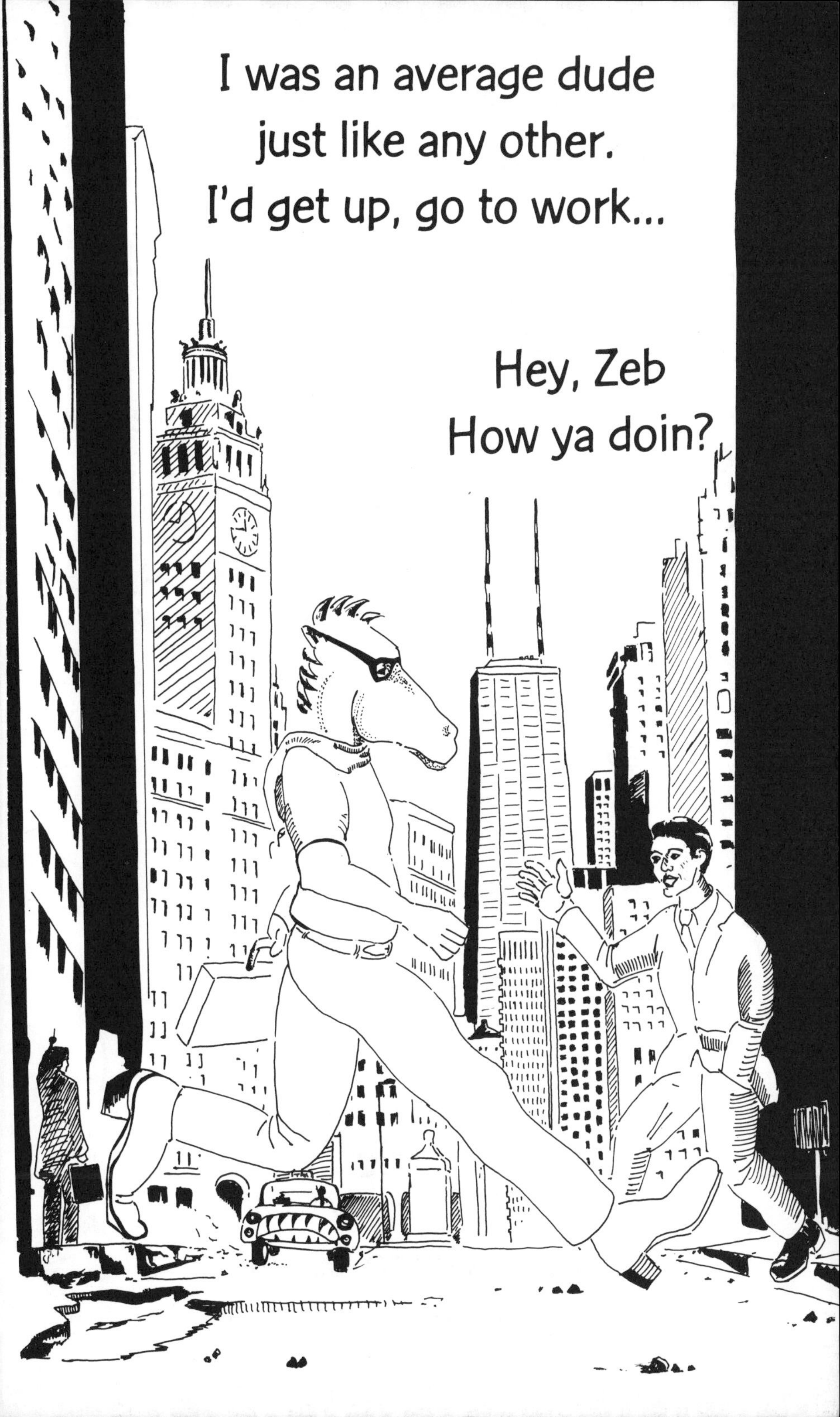
I was an average dude
just like any other.
I'd get up, go to work...
Hey, Zeb
How ya doin?

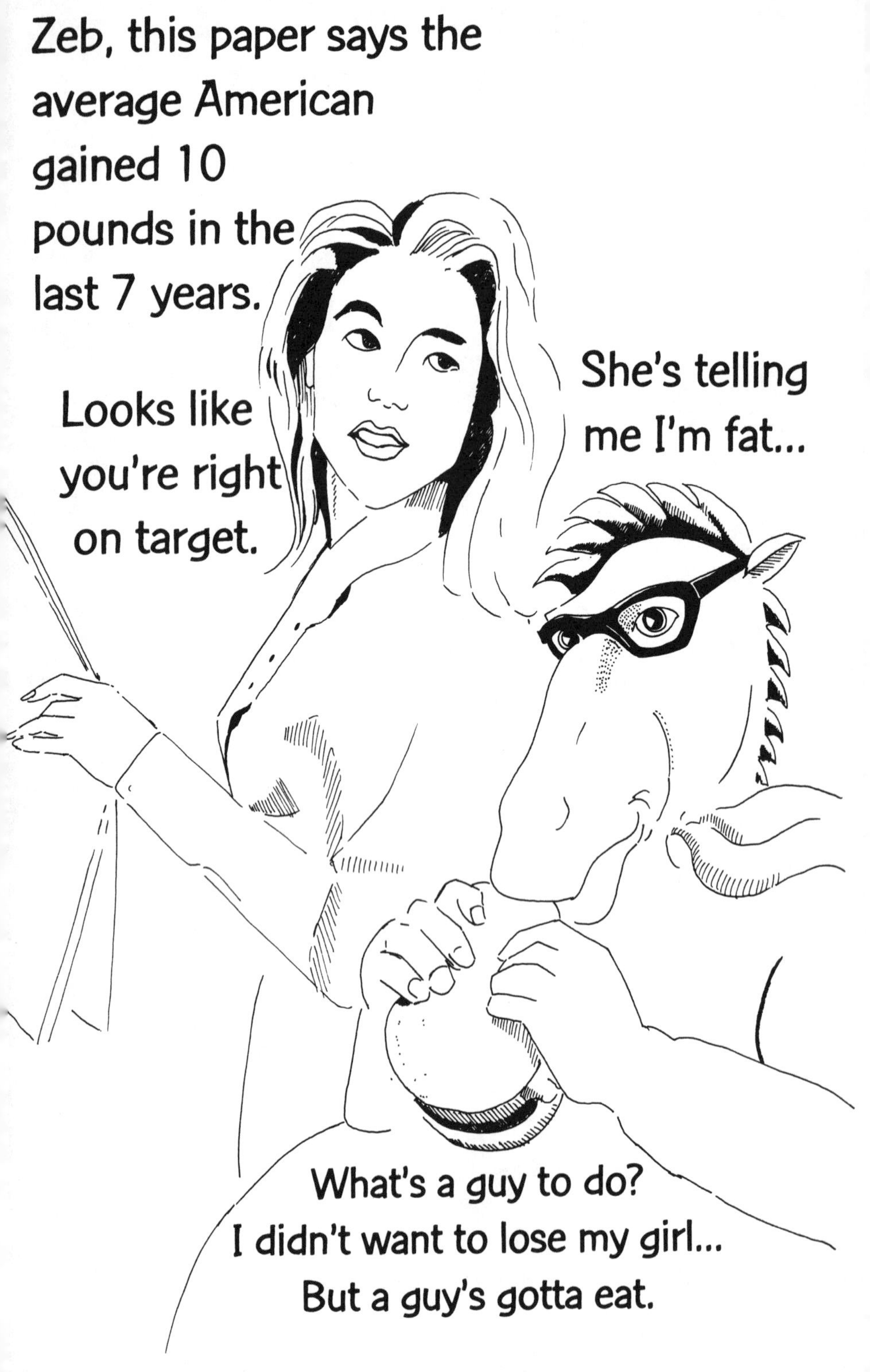
Zeb, this paper says the average American gained 10 pounds in the last 7 years.
Looks like you're right on target.
She's telling me I'm fat...
What's a guy to do? I didn't want to lose my girl... But a guy's gotta eat.

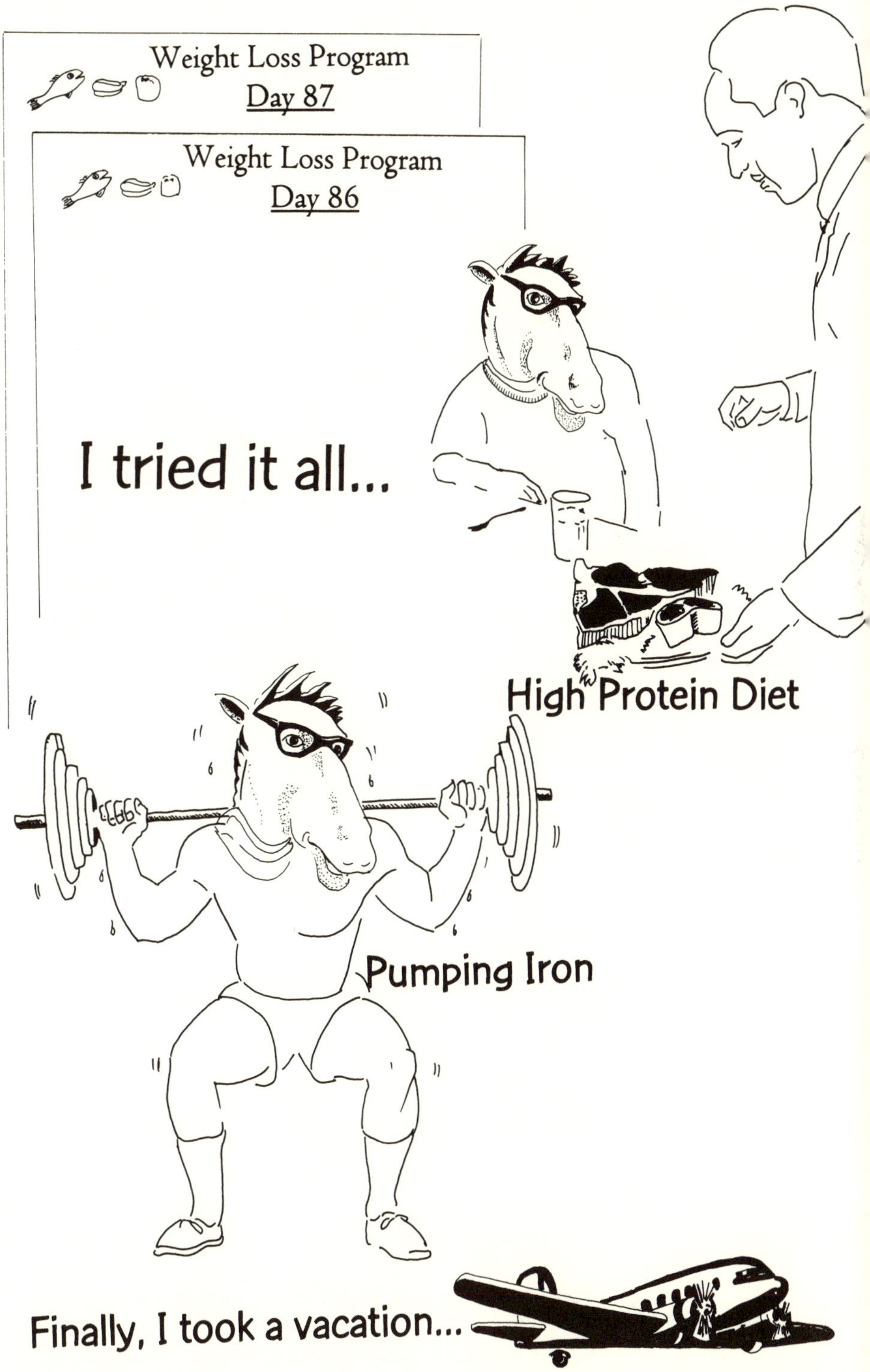
Weight Loss Program
Day 87
Weight Loss Program
Day 86
I tried it all...
High Protein Diet
Pumping Iron
Finally, I took a vacation...

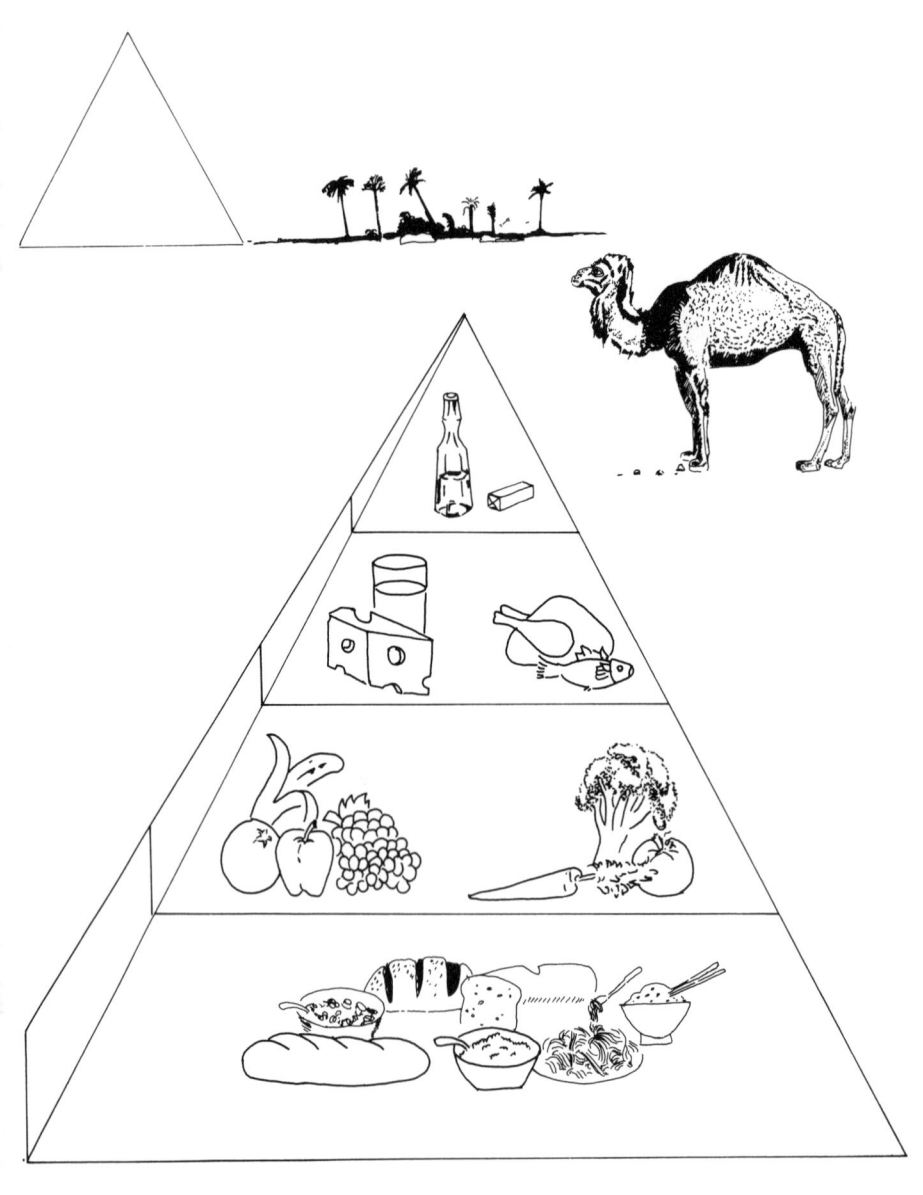

The Secret of the Pyramid

"Cut the Fat!"

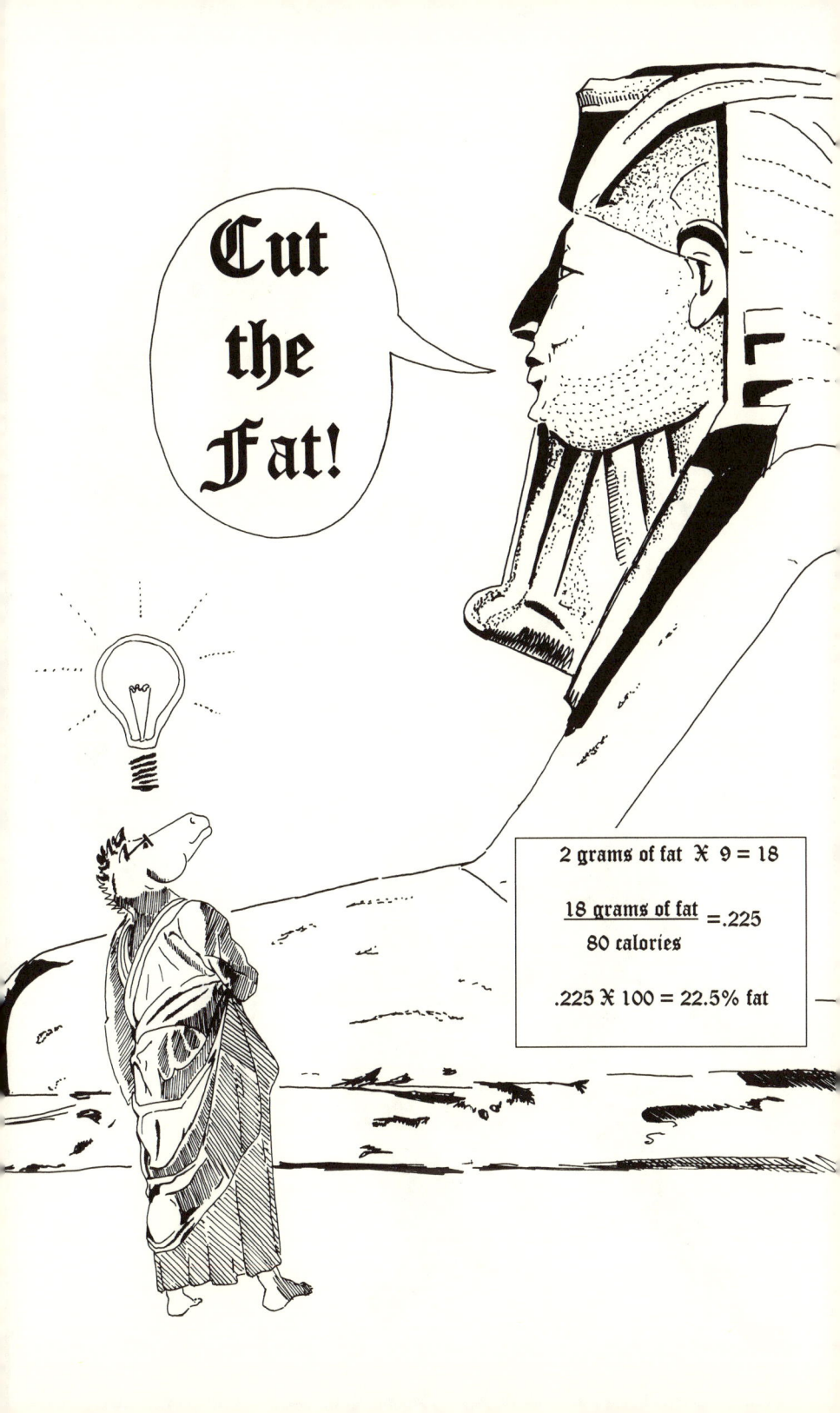

2 grams of fat ✕ 9 = 18

$$\frac{18 \text{ grams of fat}}{80 \text{ calories}} = .225$$

.225 ✕ 100 = 22.5% fat

Feelin'

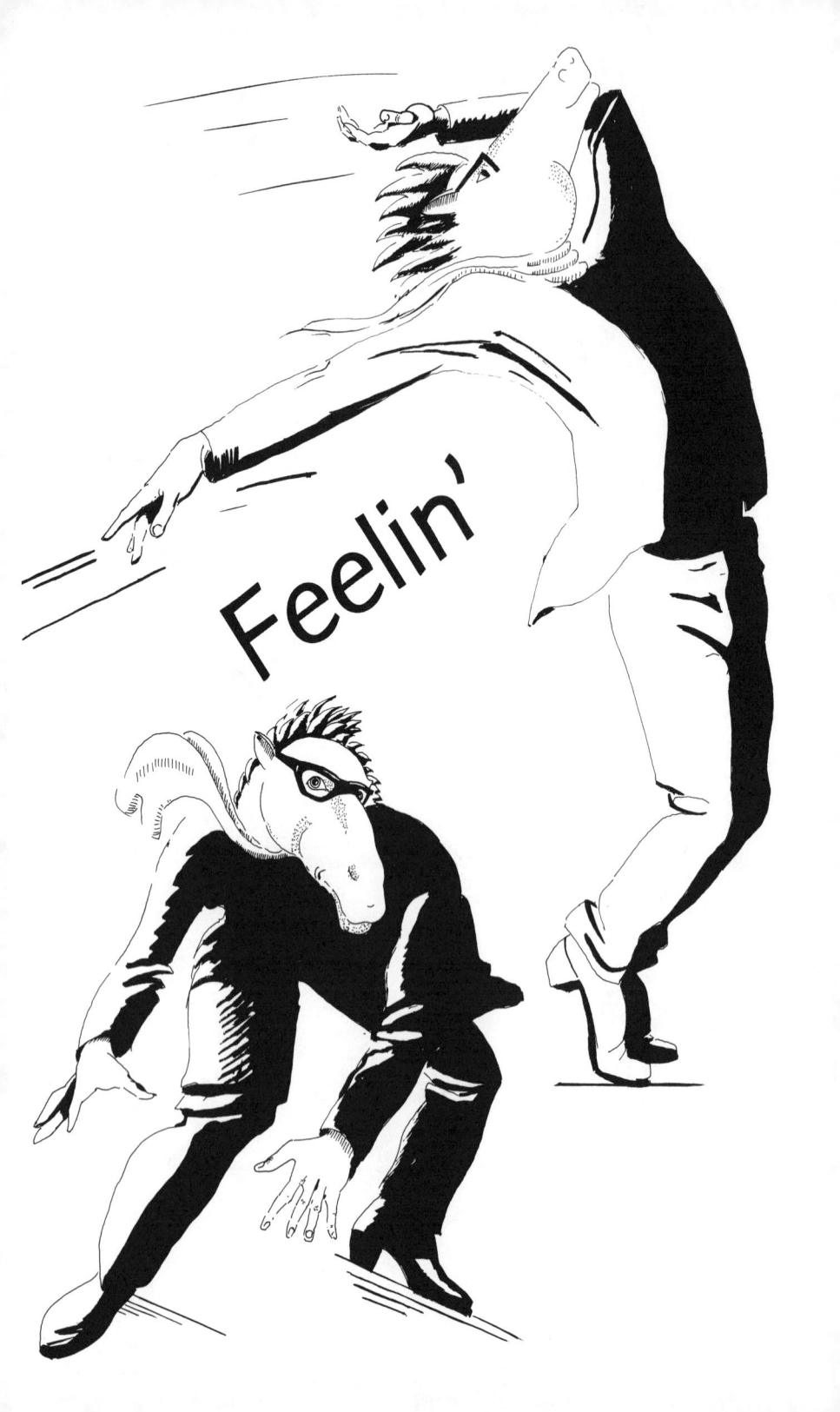

my

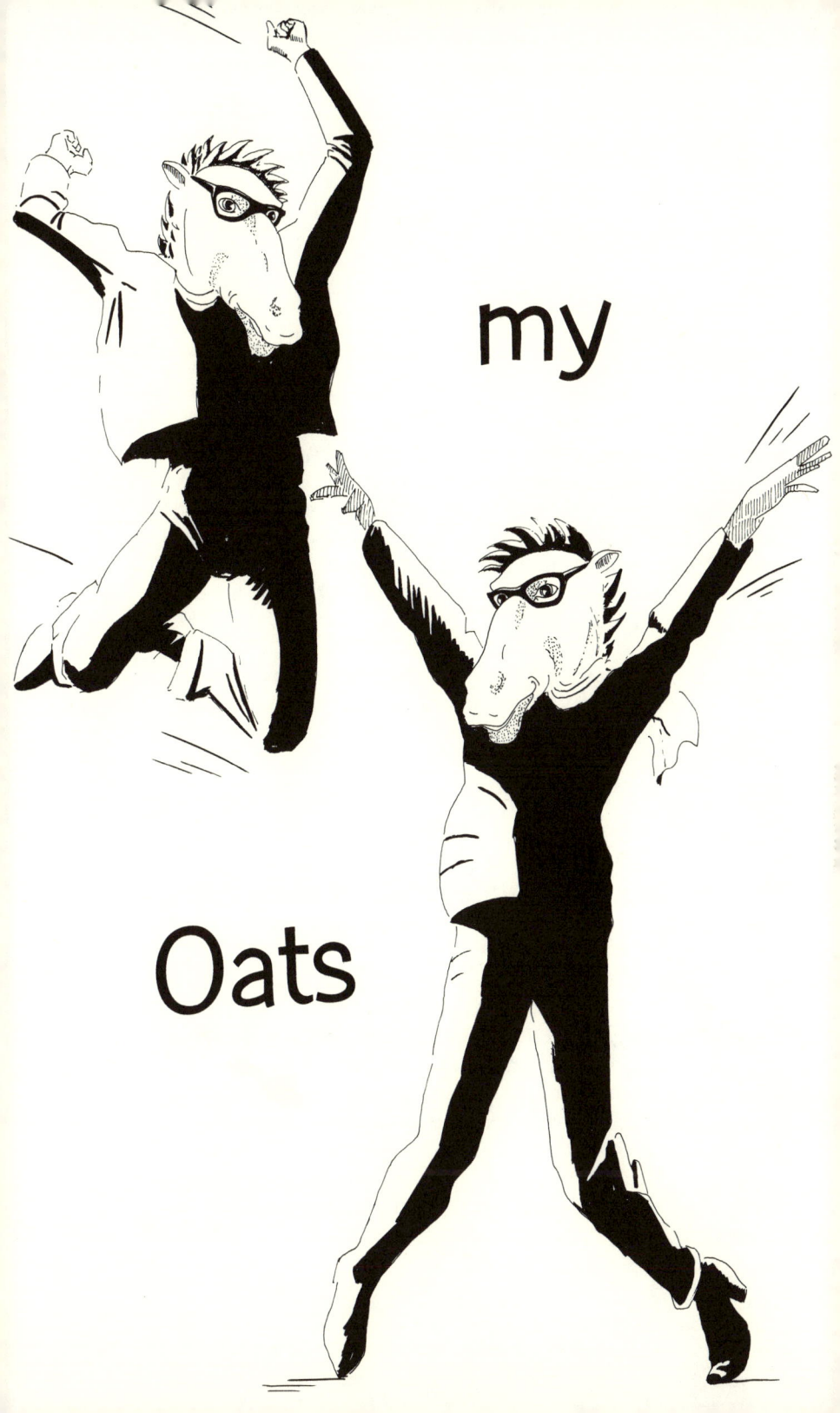

Oats

About the Recipes

"Tired blood is low-oxygen blood and low-oxygen blood is too high in fats."   *Nathan Pritikin*

Fat consciousness has exploded across America. In May 1994 the US Government regulated that all packaged food products must contain Nutrition Fact labeling. A month later the government announced a major overhaul of the public school lunch program to low fat, low sodium and healthier lunches—the first such change since 1946 when the school lunch program started.

The nutritional information is in—low fat food has exceptional health benefits. A low fat diet combined with a regular exercise program reduces heart disease, cholesterol levels, arteriosclerosis and certain cancers like breast and prostrate, as well as increases stamina and longevity.

It is in that spirit and toward that goal that these recipes were developed. Every attempt has been made to accurately gauge fat content of the recipes in this collection. Even still, you'll need to read nutrition labels: Fat content varies widely between manufacturers.

Ease of preparation: We're all stressed to the max. Many of the recipes are de-fatted and streamlined old favorites. If you have the inclination, use your homemade chicken stock in recipes calling for chicken broth. But with time at a premium, few of us have the time to get a stock pot going. Therefore, the recipes that require chicken or beef broth call for canned broth, the two most readily-available brands are approximately 14 ounces.

For the same reason we use canned beans throughout the book, but if you usually soak and cook your beans, by all means do so.

A lot of the recipes call for cooked chicken breasts. Supermarkets now carry rotisserie cooked chicken breasts and they, with skin removed, are good time-savers, albeit expensive.

Herbs and spices are ideal alternatives to fat, salt and sugar. As our collective palette grows more sophisticated due to increased restaurant dining and travel, we become more accustomed to spices and flavorings that were alien tastes just a few years ago. The home cook may easily duplicate these flavors.

We recommend that you buy your spices in bulk at the health food store. This is for several reasons: The spices are not irradiated; You can buy a large assortment in small quantities for half the price of the supermarket spice racks; and you can control freshness by buying small quantities. Save small jars to stash your spices.

In addition to a hefty reliance on herbs for flavor and spice, certain foods recur throughout. Scallions, or green onions, are used for color and crunch and require no sautéing in oil as do onions. Garlic also assumes an important role in many of the recipes. Its contribution to health is equal to its significance as a flavoring. Asiago cheese also makes a regular appearance. Asiago has a fat content of 30%—most cheeses have a fat content of 45-50%+. Asiago is less expensive than Parmesan and has a more distinct flavor so you can use less. Buy a wedge and shred it in the food processor. Place the shredded cheese in a baggy and place the baggy in a plastic bowl with lid. You will always have a supply on hand. Refrigerated, the cheese will keep up to 6 weeks.

Potatoes provide the "cream" basis for many low/no fat soups. Instant potato flakes are also a good thickener. Use the microwave oven to zap-cook a potato in minutes. (Remember to pierce the skin with a cooking fork.) Place the potato on a paper plate and cook on high for 5-6 minutes or until fork-tender.

Make your own cooking spray. A little goes a long way and the more flavorful the oil (like walnut or extra virgin olive oil), the more gusto. The family of tasteless oils like safflower, corn and canola can be punched up by adding whole chili peppers, black peppercorns and mustard seed to the oil. To make homemade cooking sprays you need to purchase spray bottles with screw-on lids and adjustable nozzles. Adjustable nozzles are necessary because oil will clog in the spray mechanism of an ordinary nozzle. These can be purchased at garden supply stores and kitchen stores. You can store the oils for up to two months in a cool, dark place.

Vinegars also impart a lot of the flavors in the book. Start with cider and wine vinegars, then add malt, rice and balsamic vinegars. Other liquids like soy sauce, Worcestershire sauce, lemon juice and Vermouth not only bestow piquancy but act as a no-fat sautéing medium.

Microwave Leftovers for lunch: Most offices have a microwave oven, cook an extra portion of whatever you make for lunch. By bringing your own lunch to work you'll save considerable money. Plus, you'll know what's in the food and you can use your lunch hour to work out at the company gym or take a walk.

Check out the Appendix for a month of menus designed to be fully balanced and tasty.

Zeb's Tips

Cheer up your refrigerator. Use the Sunday newspaper comic pages as bin liners.

Buy organic! It's good to you and the earth.

Peel peppers to remove the wax coating and superficial pesticide residue, if you don't buy organic.

Slice mushrooms with an egg slicer.

Smash ginger with a garlic press.

When cooking on the grill, spray the spatula and grill racks with cooking spray before cooking or flipping.

Save time: Buy cut-up vegetables from the supermarket salad bar for pizza, soups and stews.

Don't salt beans until after they have plumped, salt slows down the softening process.

Secret of a great bean soup: A squirt of fresh lemon juice added to the finished soup.

One tablespoon of fresh herbs equals one teaspoon of dried.

Speed up the cooking of pasta by covering the pot with a lid. When the water has come to a boil remove the lid.

For cool pasta salads: Cook pasta according to directions, then drain in a colander and run cold water over the pasta for a minute.

Double or triple the productivity of your oven, when baking a dish, also bake a couple of potatoes, or oven-roast vegetables for another use.

Roast chicken with the skin on on a rack in the roasting pan. When cooked remove the skin—the chicken will be juicy, tender, and de-fatted.

Always use non-stick cookware for sautéing, searing or browning. Buy pans from warehouse stores in packages of 3 sauté pans: 12", 10" and 8", which covers most households' needs. The pans have wooden handles and sell for less than twenty dollars for three. The non-stick surface of even the best gourmet pans will eventually wear out, so it's a good idea to buy pans in the low-end range and dispose of them after a couple of years when they wear out.

Fight salmonella. An easy and economical way to keep kitchen counters and plastic cutting boards sanitary is to keep in the kitchen a spray bottle filled with 1 part bleach and 20 parts water. Spray the surface with bleach, then dry with a sponge or paper toweling. Be sure to label the spray bottle and keep out of reach of young children.

Message to new cooks: If kitchens are alien territory to you, or if this is your first cookbook purchase, here's a list of pantry staples that seasoned cooks always have on hand.

Asiago or parmesan cheese	Garlic
Baking powder	Honey
Baking soda	Ketchup
Basil	Lemons for juice
Bay leaf	Mayonnaise
Black pepper	Mustard
Bouillon cubes	Onions
Bread crumbs	Oregano
Brown sugar	Parsley
Butter or margarine	Salt
Cayenne pepper	Soy sauce
Chili powder	Thyme
Cinnamon	Worcestershire sauce
Cloves, ground	Vanilla extract
Cocoa	Vegetable and olive oils
Cornstarch	Vinegar
Flour	

GOOD MORNING

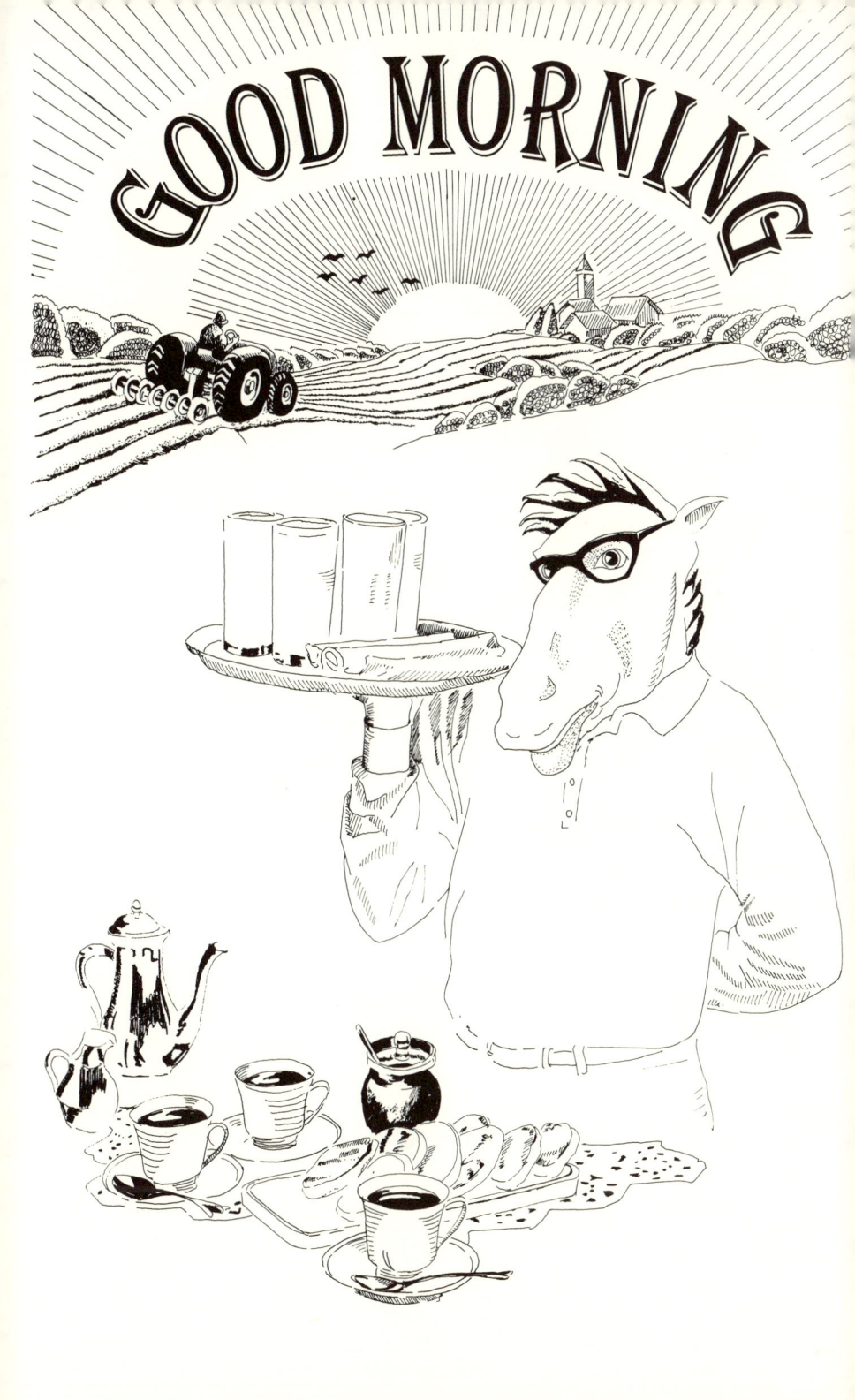

Microwave Oatmeal

That oatmeal is a horse's delight
Does follow sure as day does night.
It warms the stomach as it fills
And banishes all aches and chills.

First take a bowl of earthenware
or plastic, porcelain if you dare.
It is metal bowls on which we frown
Your microwave will melt it down.

In this bowl a banana mash
and after it some water splash.
Add oats to halfway to the top
And as topping, raisins plop.

Five minutes in a microwave
for b'fast that a king could crave.
If he but knew the warm pleasure
Above his gold his oats he'd treasure.

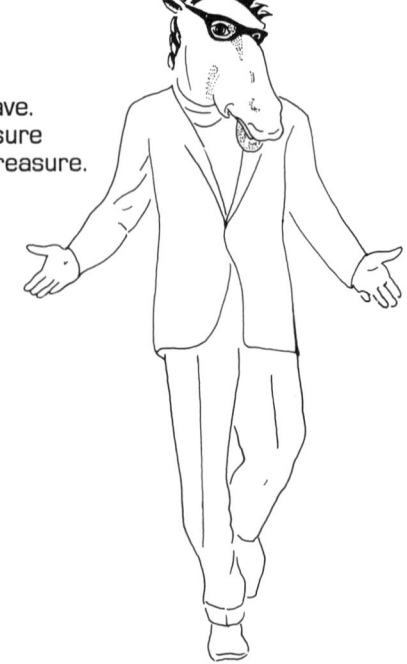

Blueberry Muffins

Makes 12 muffins
0 grams per serving

Everybody's favorite muffin. Frozen blueberries may be substituted for fresh. Use restraint when blending the liquid and dry ingredients, mix just to combine. For best results, have the egg whites and yogurt at room temperature.

   2 cups flour
   1 Tbs baking powder
   ½ tsp salt
   1 ½ cups fresh blueberries
   4 egg whites
   ½ cup sugar
   1 ½ cups plain nonfat yogurt
   1 tsp vanilla
   2 Tbs sugar
   1 tsp cinnamon

Preheat oven to 400°. Fill muffin tin with paper liners. In a large bowl, sift together the first three ingredients. Add blueberries and gently coat them with the flour mixture.

In a separate bowl, beat egg whites with an electric mixer at high speed until stiff. Add ½ cup sugar, yogurt and vanilla. Continue to beat for about 30 seconds. Add the yogurt mixture to the dry ingredients. With a spatula, use a lifting motion to mix the batter. Do not overmix. Spoon the batter into the prepared muffin tins.

In a small bowl, combine together the remaining sugar and cinnamon. Sprinkle the mixture over the muffins and bake for 20 minutes.

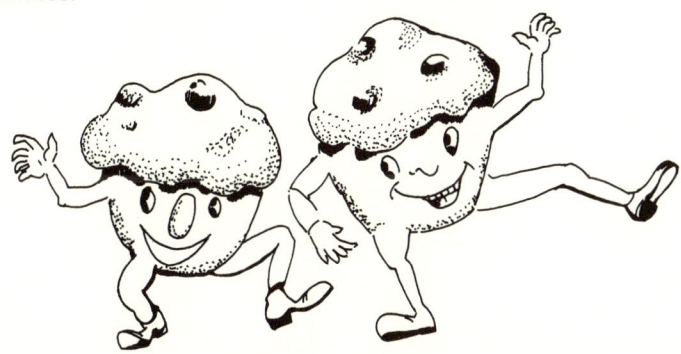

Granola

Serves 12
2.3 grams per serving

Start the day right. Granola, skim milk, and fresh fruit will fire you up to meet the challenges of a new day. Or use a spoonful or two as a topping on nonfat frozen yogurt.

½ cup frozen apple juice concentrate, thawed
¼ cup honey
1 Tbs vanilla
3 cups rolled oats
½ cup wheat germ
1 Tbs cinnamon
1 tsp ground nutmeg (optional)
1 cup lightly packed flaked coconut
1 cup raisins

Preheat oven to 275°. In a small bowl, mix together apple juice concentrate, honey and vanilla. In a large bowl, combine the oats, wheat germ, cinnamon and ground nutmeg (if desired). Stir the liquid ingredients into the dry ingredients; break up large clumps.

Spread the granola onto a large baking sheet and bake for 30 minutes, turning with a spatula halfway through. Stir in the coconut and bake for an additional 30 minutes, until crunchy and lightly browned.

Remove from the oven. Cool. Toss in the raisins. Store in an airtight container in the refrigerator for up to a month.

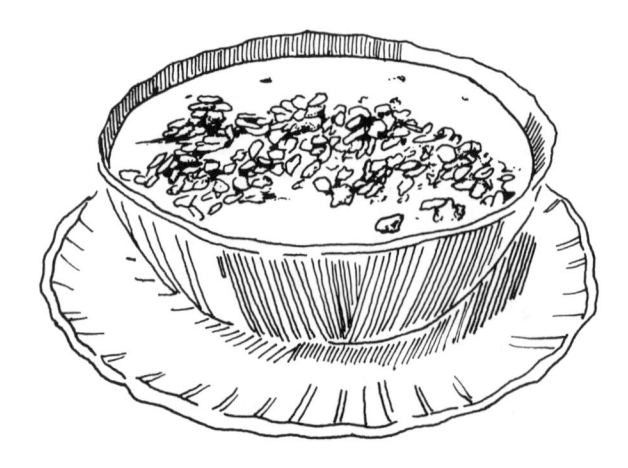

Failproof Popovers

Makes 6 popovers
1.5 grams per serving

1 cup skim milk
1 cup unsifted flour
¼ tsp salt
2 egg whites and 1 egg yolk, unbeaten
1 tsp butter

Place milk, flour, salt and eggs in a mixing bowl. Stir with a spoon until flour is moist. Mixture will be lumpy. Grease six cold glass custard cups with butter. Fill with batter and put in cold oven. Set oven at 450° and bake for 10 minutes. Turn heat down to 350°. Bake 35 minutes. Do not open oven door!

Serve immediately with jam.

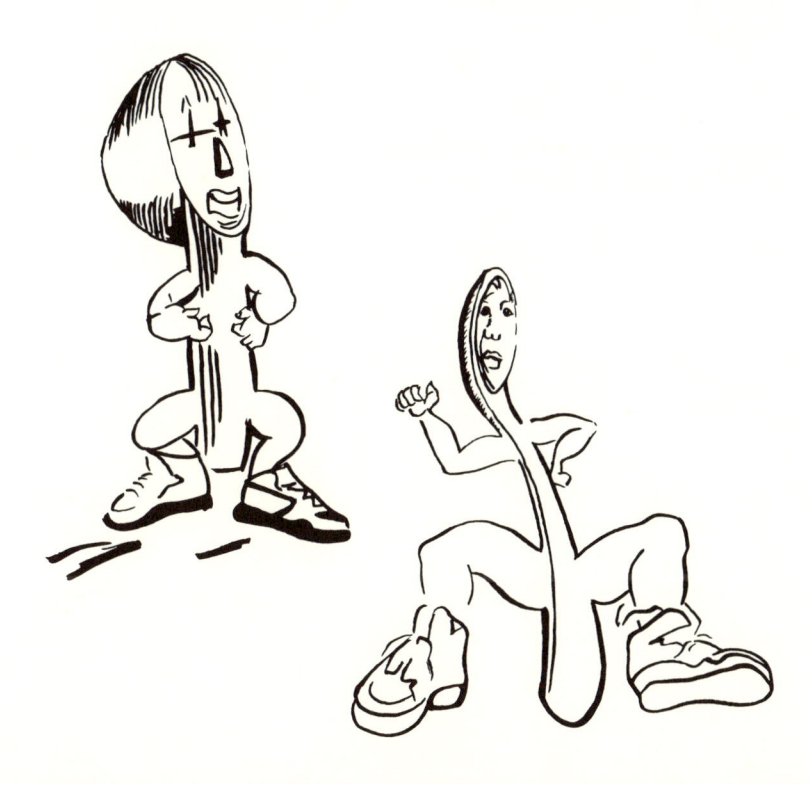

Yogurt and Fruit

Serves 1-2
0 grams per serving

A bowl of fresh fruit smothered in fruit-flavored nonfat yogurt is a gratifying way to greet the day. And it appeals to the senses—cheerful pink strawberry yogurt, the crunch of an apple, the aromas of sliced oranges, the smoothness of a ripe banana—all combined with the satisfying knowledge that you're making a healthy dent in the 5-6 fresh fruits recommended daily for good nutrition. Complete your fruit bowl with toast and jam, or top with granola (see recipe page 18).

   Small carton fruit-flavored nonfat yogurt
   1 apple, peeled, cored and sliced in chunks
   1 orange, peeled and sectioned
   1 ripe banana, sliced
   Fruits in season: Berries, melons, tropical fruits, etc.

Stir yogurt and fruits together into a bowl. Top with granola, if desired.

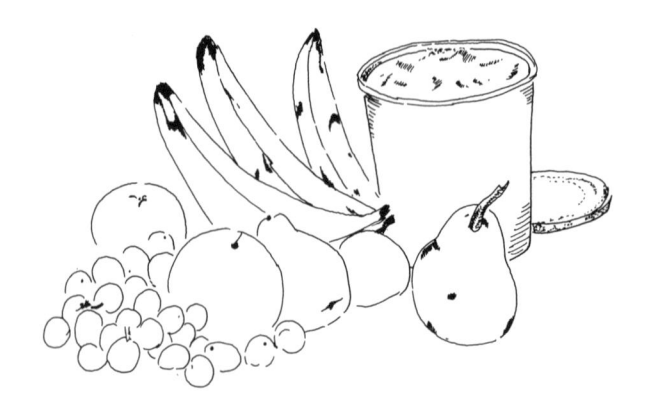

Breakfast Cake

Serves 8
2.5 grams per serving

A delicious cake that can be popped in the oven in 10 minutes' time.

    1 whole egg and 1 egg white
    ¼ cup skim milk
    ½ cup sugar
    1½ cups flour
    ½ tsp salt
    ¼ tsp cinnamon
    ¼ tsp ground cloves
    2 apples, peeled, cored and sliced
    2 pears, peeled, cored and sliced
    1 Tbs grated lemon or orange peel
    ¼ cup sliced almonds

Preheat oven to 350°. Beat the eggs in a large bowl. Add milk, then sugar, continuing to beat until frothy. Add flour, salt, cinnamon and cloves, mixing well. The batter will be thick. Add the fruit and lemon peel, stirring until the fruit is coated.

Spoon the batter into a 9" greased cake pan. Top with almonds and bake the cake for 40 minutes or until a wooden pick inserted in the middle comes out clean.

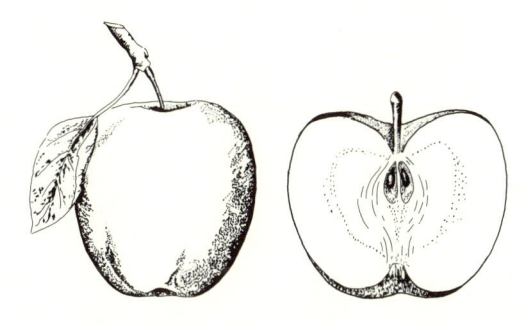

Southwestern Eggs

Serves 4
5.5 grams per serving

Ideal for brunch or lunch. A meal in minutes.

    1 cup nonfat refried beans
    4 large eggs
    4 corn tortillas
    Salsa (recipes begin on page 44)

Heat the refried beans in a covered dish in the microwave or in the oven. Poach the eggs in the microwave* or on the stove. Place the tortillas on a baking sheet and warm for 3-5 minutes. Spread ¼ cup refried beans on a tortilla. Place a poached egg over the beans and 1-2 Tbs salsa over the eggs. Repeat with the other three tortillas.

* To poach eggs in the microwave: Put 2 cups hot tap water in a microwave-safe bowl and boil at high for 5-6 minutes. Break eggs onto a plate, puncturing the yolk. Swirl boiling water with a spoon, carefully slip in eggs. Cover. Microwave at medium for one minute per egg, 45 seconds per egg for more than one egg. Let eggs stand in water for a few minutes.

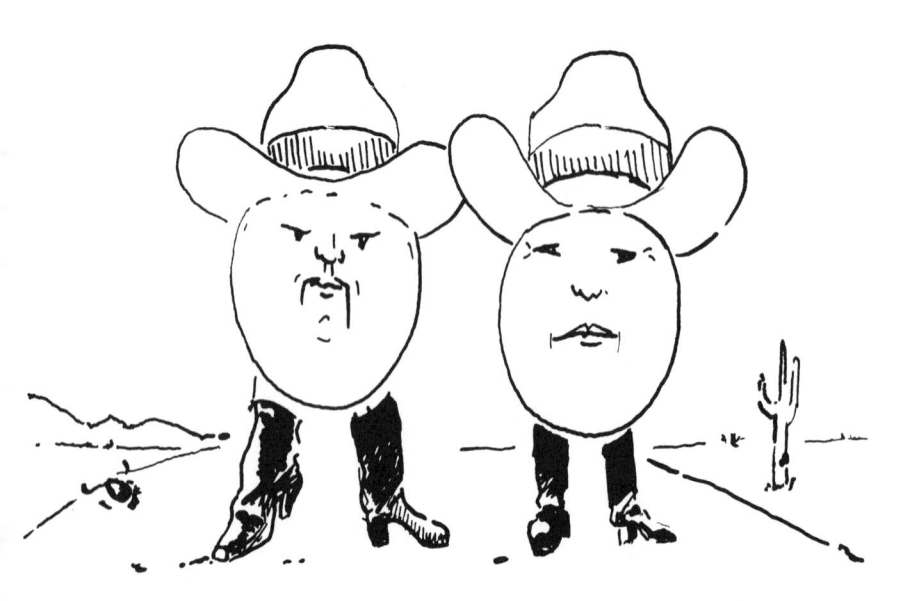

Bran Muffins

Makes 12 muffins
3 grams per serving

The word of the day: Salubrious. That's what these hearty muffins are—wholesome, nutritious and low fat.

1 cup 100% bran cereal (not flakes)
1 large egg, beaten
1 cup ripe bananas, mashed
¾ cup raisins
¾ cup skim milk
2 Tbs oil
1 cup flour
¼ cup sugar
1 Tbs baking powder
½ tsp. cinnamon
¼ tsp salt

Preheat oven to 400°. Put paper liners in a muffin tin, or spray with cooking spray. Combine first six ingredients in a bowl. Stir lightly and let stand for about 10 minutes.

Sift the remaining ingredients in a medium bowl. Stir the dry ingredients into the banana mixture until just combined—do not overstir. Spoon batter into a muffin tin. Bake for 20 minutes, or until a toothpick inserted in center of muffin comes out clean.

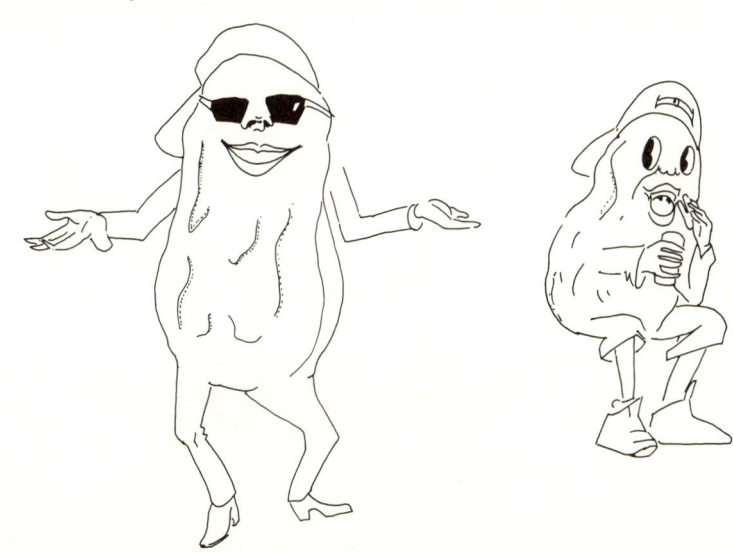

Eggs Sardou

Serves 4
7.5 grams per serving

    1 10 oz. package frozen creamed spinach
    4 eggs
    2 English muffins, split in half

Heat creamed spinach according to package directions. Poach the eggs in a boiling water bath on the stove or in the microwave (see method on page 22). Toast the English muffins.

Place 1 poached egg on each muffin half. Spoon ¼ portion creamed spinach over each egg. Serve at once.

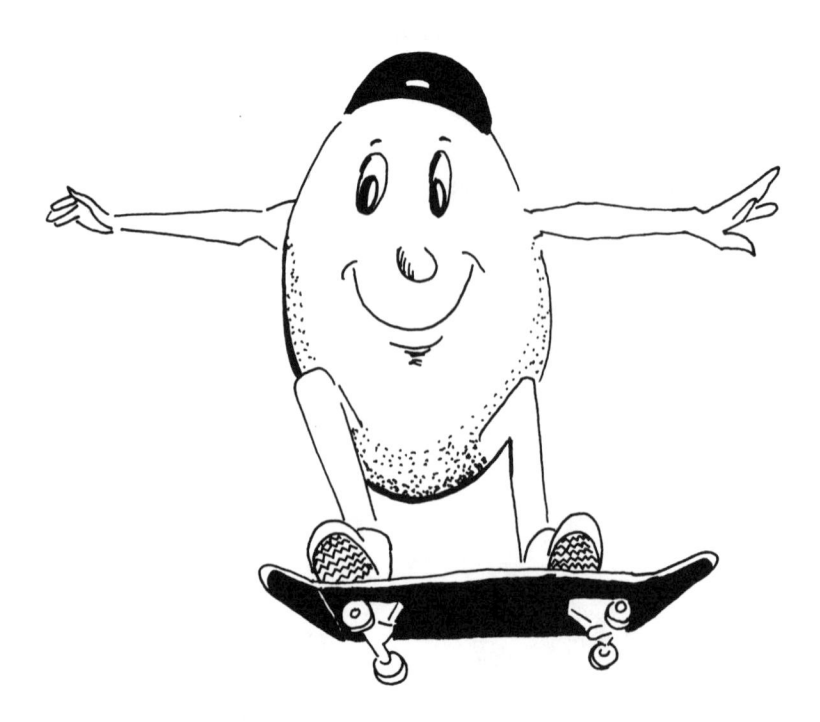

Frittata

Serves 4
8.5 grams per serving

Frittata...today's answer to quiche. With the odd bits of cooked veggies in the fridge, you can whip up a lovely brunch in minutes. Let the seasons be your inspiration—summer's tomato and basil bounty makes a glorious frittata; in autumn, team spinach and mushroom with red pepper; in winter, we like braised leek; and in spring, tender asparagus. But no matter which vegetable combinations you use, always start with cooked potatoes and take it from there....

4 eggs
2 egg whites
¾ cup skim milk
¼ tsp salt and pepper
1 cup boiled or baked potatoes, sliced
8 fresh basil leaves, or ½ tsp dried
2 scallions, chopped
½ cup shredded cheese
cooking spray

Any of the following vegetables:
½ cup sliced mushrooms (sautéed in wine)
1 cup fresh spinach leaves
½ cup green or red pepper, chopped
6 asparagus spears, cooked and diced *or* small can, drained
2 tomatoes, sliced thin

Preheat oven to 350°. Place eggs and egg whites in a medium bowl and whisk until frothy. Add milk, salt and pepper to eggs and stir well to combine. Add potatoes and vegetables (except tomatoes), stirring to coat with egg mixture.

Spray an 8" x 8" baking dish with cooking spray. Pour the egg-vegetable mixture into the pan. Top with basil, tomatoes, scallions and cheese. Bake for 35 minutes until set and lightly browned on top.

Raisin Bread

Makes 1 loaf
less than 1 gram per serving

No need to knead.

    1 cup raisins
    1 cup water
    1 cup All Bran cereal
    ½ cup sugar
    ½ cup oatmeal
    1 cup whole wheat flour
    1 Tbs baking soda
    ¼ tsp salt
    1 cup buttermilk
    veg oil spray

Preheat oven to 350°. Simmer the raisins in the water in a small pan for 5 minutes. Drain the water from the raisins.

Combine the dry ingredients in a large bowl. Add the buttermilk and raisins. Mix with a large spoon. With your hands, shape the dough into a loaf. Place the dough into a loaf pan sprayed with cooking spray.

Bake for 35-40 minutes.

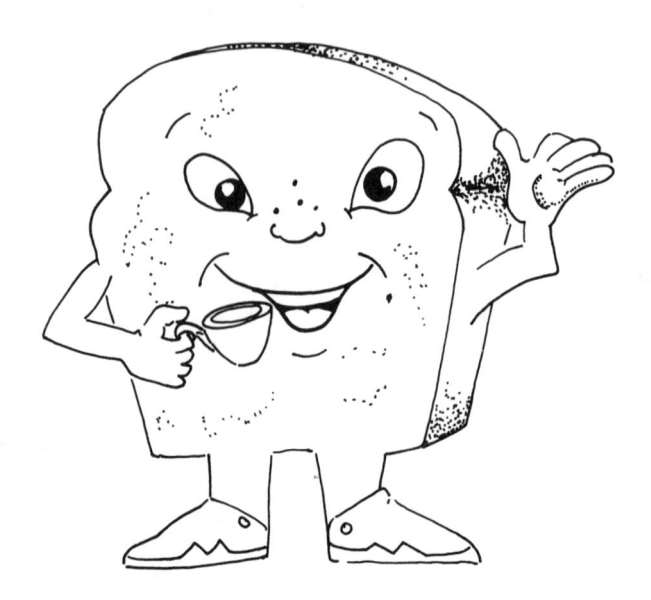

STARTERS

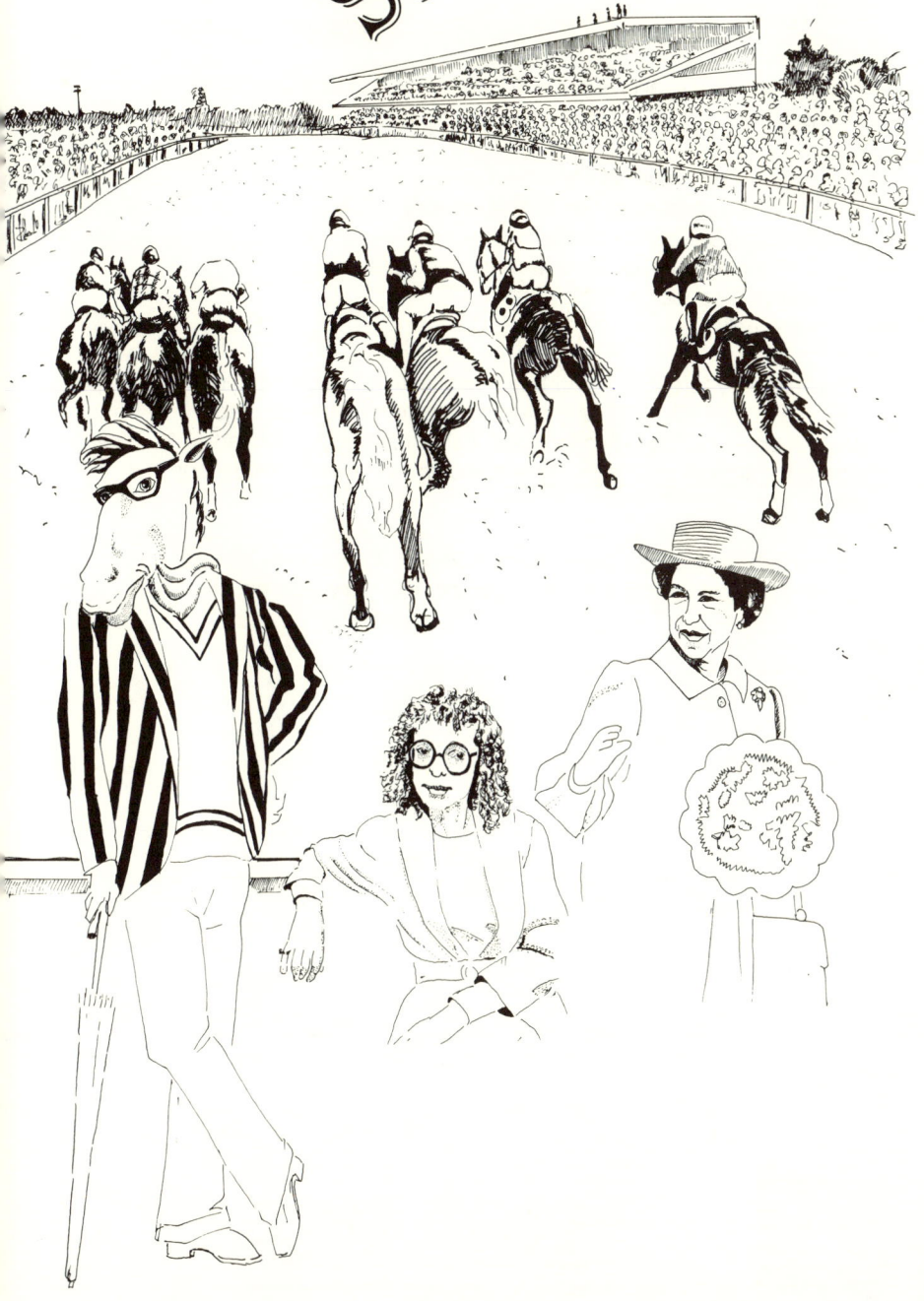

Stuffed Cherry Tomatoes

Makes 36 appetizers
Trace grams per 6 appetizers

A quick and easy party yummy, makes an attractive Christmas canapé tray.

- 1 pint cherry tomatoes
- 1 15-oz carton nonfat ricotta cheese
- 1-2 tsp balsamic vinegar
- 3 Tbs finely-chopped fresh basil or parsley
- salt and pepper, to taste
- skim milk

Wash cherry tomatoes. With a sharp knife, slice the cherry tomatoes in half. Carefully scoop out the pulp and seeds, discard. Mix together ricotta, vinegar, basil, salt and pepper. Add small amounts of skim milk, stirring until the mixture is of creamy consistency.

Fill tomato halves with the cheese mixture. Arrange on a plate. Cover with plastic wrap and refrigerate until serving time.

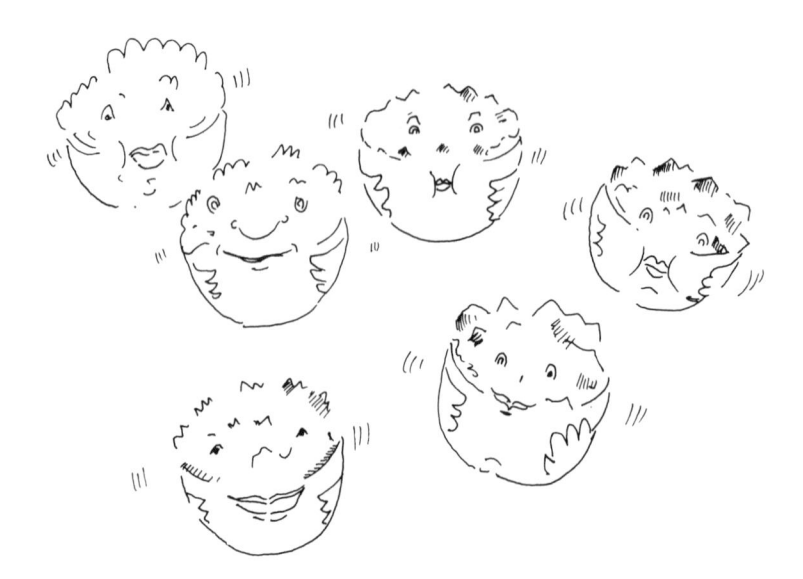

Roquefort 'Shrooms

Makes 30 appetizers
1.2 grams per appetizer

Just what we like, a nibble that costs only about one gram each. These can be prepared in advance, refrigerated, then popped under the broiler prior to serving.

> 30 medium mushrooms, well cleaned
> 4 oz Roquefort cheese
> 1 cup seasoned bread crumbs
> ¼ cup minced shallots
> 2 Tbs dry sherry or brandy
> cooking spray
> chopped parsley as a garnish

Remove stems from the mushrooms. Mince the stems. Combine the Roquefort, bread crumbs, minced mushroom stems and shallots. Mix well. Stir in sherry or brandy and mix well again.

Stuff each mushroom cap with a mound of the filling. Spray a baking sheet with cooking spray. Place the mushrooms on the baking sheet. Broil for about 5 minutes, but keep an eye on it!—don't let the 'shrooms burn.

Garnish with parsley and serve hot.

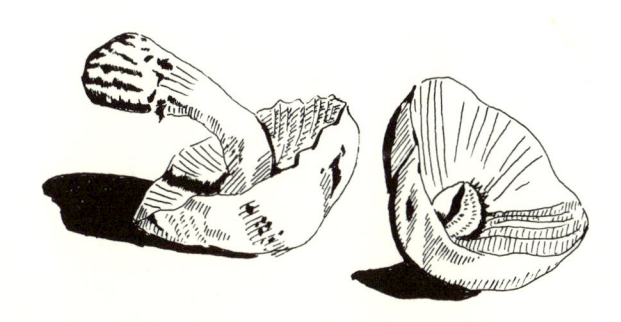

Scare Away Werewolves Roasted Garlic

Serves 2-3
Trace grams per serving

Garlic, when roasted, loses its well-known undesirable traits, resulting in a mild and buttery paste that's a delicious appetizer when spread over crackers or thin French bread.

    2-3 plump garlic bulbs
    1 tsp olive oil

Select only the freshest, plumpest bulbs. Preheat oven to 350°. Measure oil into small baking dish. Swirl garlic bulbs in the oil and arrange root side down in the dish. Bake for 30-45 minutes, or until the garlic is soft.

For a spread: Squeeze the garlic into a small ramekin. Place in the center of a plate surrounded by bread or crackers.

For an appetizer: Place each bulb on a small plate surrounded by thinly-sliced French bread.

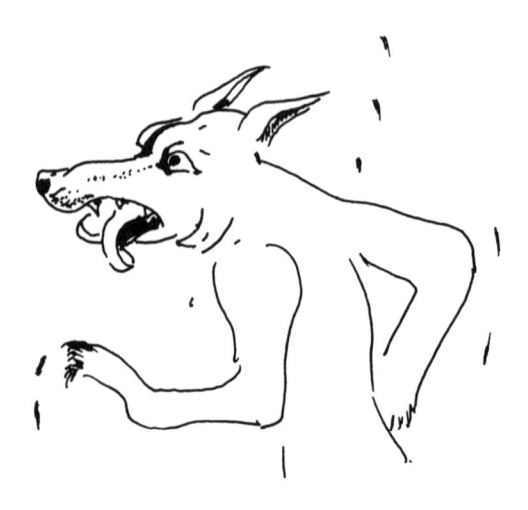

Tapenade

Makes ¾ cup
1 gram per ¼ cup serving

Typically, tapenade is high fat heaven: Black olives, anchovy paste, and capers swimming in olive oil, with a dangerous coronary corollary—an astronomical sodium content. This low fat variation is tasty without the excess salt of the traditional tapenade. A unique appetizer.

    1 bulb roasted garlic (see previous recipe)
    1 3¼-oz can water-packed tuna, drained
    3-4 Tbs capers
    fresh ground pepper
    lemon

Squeeze garlic from skins and place in the work bowl of a food processor. Add the remaining ingredients and pulse until ingredients are combined. If too dry, add a squeeze of lemon. Serve on toast rounds.

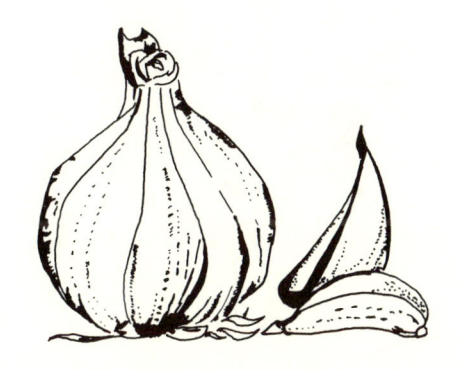

Oven-crisped Corn Chips

Makes 72 chips
Trace grams per 6 chips

Nonfat and low-fat corn chips can be purchased at most health food stores, but they are very easy to make at home and cheaper! Fat content of corn tortillas varies from brand to brand. Read package labels for nonfat corn tortillas.

    1 dozen corn tortillas
    cooking spray
    chili powder or garlic powder (optional)

Preheat oven to 350°. Lightly spray both sides of the tortillas with cooking spray. Sprinkle optional chili or garlic powder on the tortillas.

Slice each tortilla into 6 pie-shaped wedges and arrange on a nonstick cookie sheet. Prepare in two batches. Bake in preheated oven for 5 minutes or until chips begin to curl. Shake the pan and continue to bake until lightly browned. Serve immediately with frijomole or mock guac.

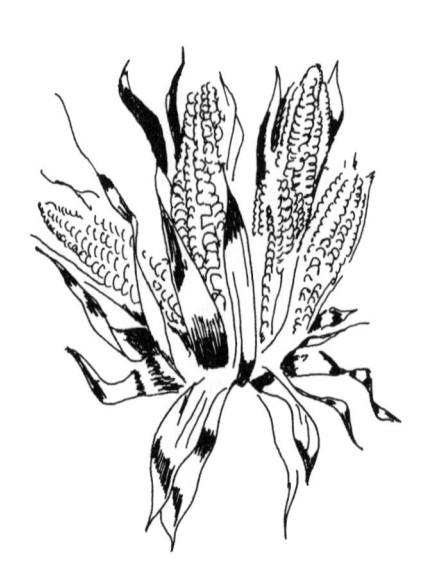

Mock Guac

Serves 6
Trace grams per serving

The average (half-pound) avocado weighs in at 30 grams of fat. Double that for guacamole and the fat count zooms off the charts. This version, made with frozen green peas, not only contains a mere trace of fat, but also retains its lovely green color. For a variation, add ripe tomato chunks to the guac.

½ cup fresh cilantro
2 garlic cloves
chili pepper flakes, to taste
1 ½ tsp powdered cumin
1 pound frozen green peas, thawed and drained
¼ cup fresh lemon or lime juice
salt and Tabasco, to taste
¼ cup diced onion
1 ripe tomato, cut in chunks (optional)
2 green onions, chopped for garnish

Put the cilantro, garlic, pepper flakes and cumin in a food processor or blender. Pulse until cilantro is minced. Add peas and lemon or lime juice and blend until peas are almost smooth. Check seasonings, adding salt and Tabasco to taste.

Spoon mock guac into a serving bowl and stir in the diced onions and tomatoes, if desired. Garnish with scallions.

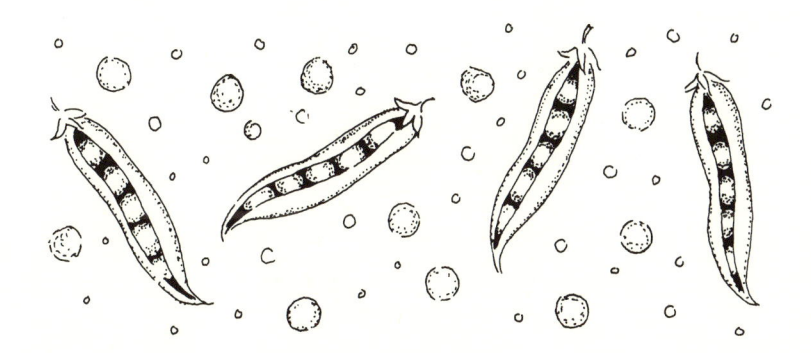

Frijomole

Makes 1½ cups
1.7 grams per ¼ cup

1 medium onion, chopped
2 tsps olive oil
1 16-oz can fat-free refried beans
2 cloves garlic, minced
2 scallions, chopped
1 chili pepper, seeded and diced
2 Tbs lime juice
1 large tomato, skinned and chopped
½ tsp Tabasco, or to taste
salt, to taste

Sauté the onion with the oil in a nonstick pan. Cook until the onion is translucent.

In a medium mixing bowl, add the beans, cooked onion, minced garlic, scallions, chili pepper and lime juice. Stir carefully to incorporate the ingredients into the beans. Season to taste with salt and Tabasco. When the mixture is smooth, fold in the chopped tomatoes.

Serve with oven-crisped corn chips (page 32).

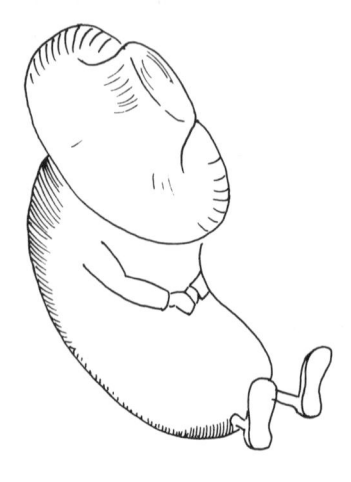

Jalapeño Dip

Makes 1 cup
2 grams per ¼ cup

A good marriage of flavors. The intrepid chili pepper lover will make this dip with two jalapeños.

    1 jalapeño pepper
    ¾ cup nonfat plain yogurt
    ¼ cup sour half-and-half
    2 tsp lime juice
    1 tsp chili powder
    ¼ tsp salt

Wearing rubber gloves, stem and seed the jalapeño, then mince it finely. Blend the minced pepper with the other ingredients in a dip bowl. Chill for a couple of hours and serve with chips or cut-up vegetables.

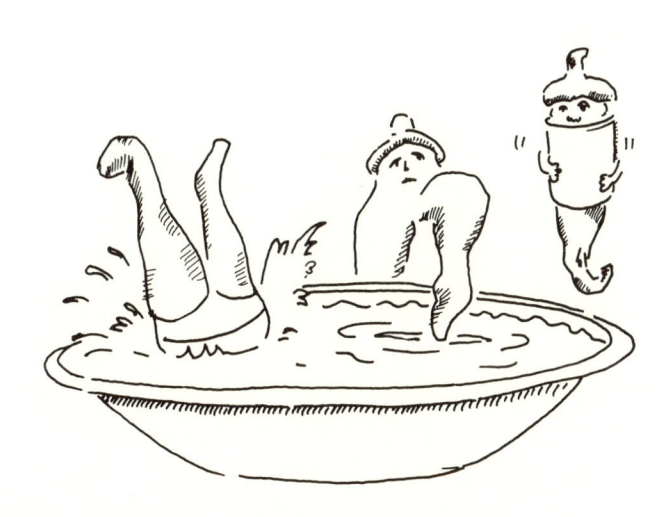

Ragin' Cajun Popcorn

Serves 4
1.5 grams per serving

Make your own! Put 1/3 cup corn kernels in a brown paper bag. (A sandwich bag is the perfect size.) Fold over twice. Microwave on high for approximately 3 minutes. You now have air-popped popcorn. But the problem with air-popped popcorn is that it tastes like packing material. Our solution is to give the popcorn a couple of blasts of cooking spray—the salt, spices and cheese will stick to the popcorn and flavor it.

> air-popped or fat-free microwave popcorn
> butter-flavored cooking spray
> 4 Tbs grated parmesan
> salt
> onion powder
> cayenne pepper
> chili powder or curry powder (but not both!)
> garlic powder

Spray popped popcorn lightly with cooking spray. Add cheese and the above seasonings, to taste. Toss to blend ingredients.

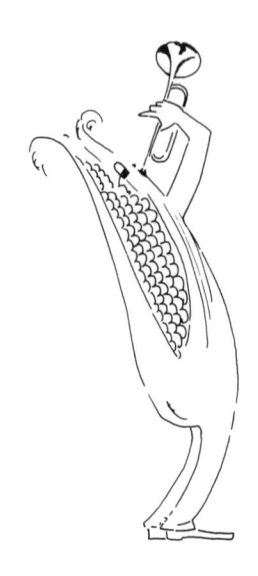

Nutty Beans

Makes 10 handsful
1 gram per handful

Next time the game's on, grab a handful of these crunchy "nuts"!

    1 19-oz can garbanzo beans
    onion powder
    cayenne pepper (to taste)
    cooking spray

Heat oven to 350°. Rinse and drain the beans. Spray a baking sheet with cooking spray. Arrange the beans in a single layer on the baking sheet. Season with onion powder and careful dashes of cayenne.

Bake for 50-60 minutes until the beans are crisped and lightly browned.

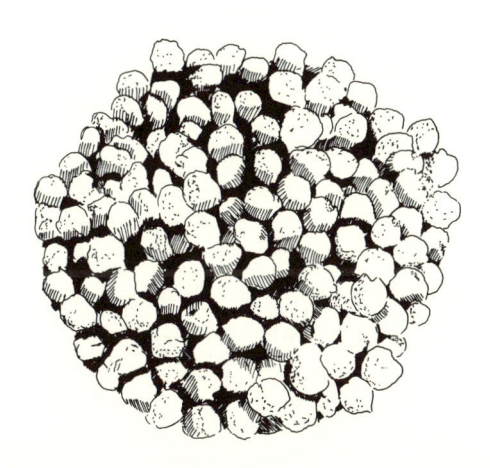

Shrimp-Cucumber Dip

Makes 2+ cups
0.6 grams total per ¼ cup

1 cup cucumber, peeled, seeded and chopped fine
2 Tbs chopped onion (or scallion)
1 tsp horseradish
1 cup 2% creamed cottage cheese
2 Tbs tarragon vinegar
¼ lb. cooked shrimp, or a 4½-oz can, drained

In a small bowl place all the ingredients except the shrimp.

Beat with a whisk until smooth. Cut the shrimp into small pieces. Add to the mixture and blend well. Cover and refrigerate until serving.

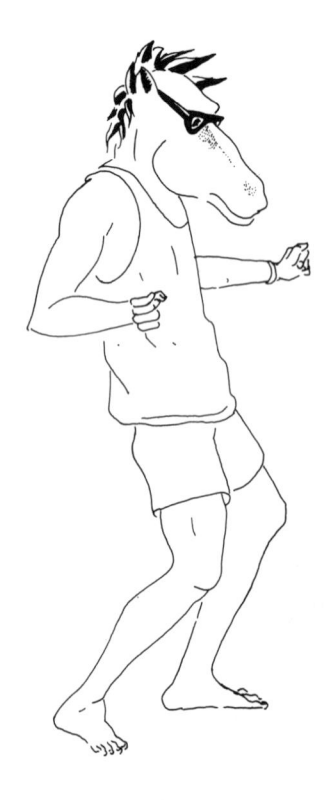

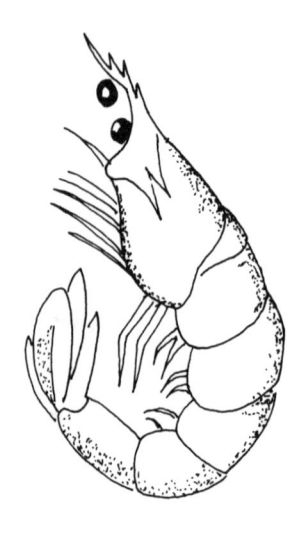

Grilled Clams

4 grams per dozen

A hot summer's afternoon...a crowd of guests waiting for barbecue. Grilled clams, served before the serious eating begins, are a perfect (and perfectly simple) appetizer. You must remember this: Chuck out any uncooked clams that are open and any cooked clams that remain closed.

> 3-4 clams—little necks, cherrystones, etc.—per person
> lemon wedges
> dash hot pepper sauce

Scrub the clams of seaweed and grit. Keep cold.

Arrange the clams on a hot grill. Cover grill. Once the clams have opened (2–3 minutes), they are ready for serving. Sprinkle lemon juice and a dash of hot pepper sauce on the clams.

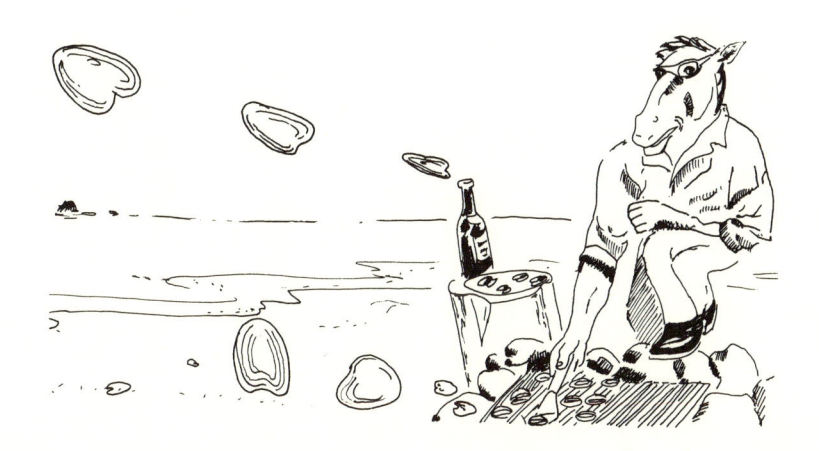

Herbed Crostini

Makes 12 crostini
2.1 grams per crostini

Good for snacking, but for a dramatic party tray, fan the crostini around a low-fat dip. You'll need two baking sheets of the same size to bake the crostini.

    1 baguette (16" loaf French bread)
    1 Tbs olive oil
    ¼ - ½ tsp garlic powder
    ½ tsp crushed rosemary
    1 tsp dried basil
    salt and pepper, to taste

Preheat oven to 350°. Cut the bread lengthwise into 4 pieces. Cut each piece into 3 long spears. You will have 12 crostini. Brush each crostini with oil, and sprinkle with remaining ingredients.

Arrange the crostini on a baking sheet. Set another baking sheet over it and bake for 15 minutes. With oven mitts, grasp both baking sheets together and flip the baking sheets. Bake for about 15 minutes more, or until lightly browned. Cool. The crostini will keep for a week in an airtight container.

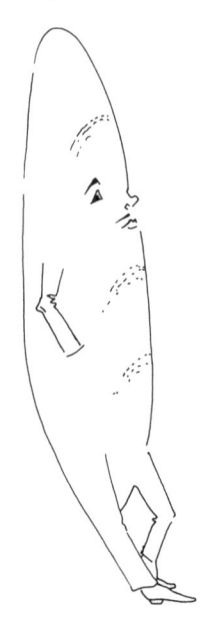

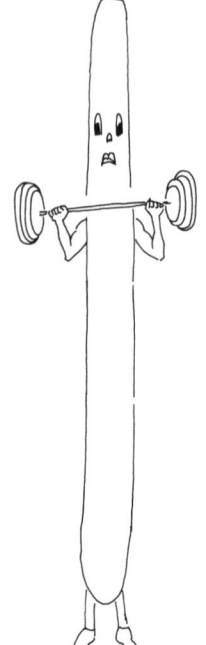

Cannellini Roll-ups

Makes 15 canapés
1.3 grams per canapé

1 19-oz can cannellini beans (Italian white beans), drained
1 clove garlic, minced
1 tsp rosemary, crushed
¼ tsp salt, or to taste
dash pepper
3 flour tortillas
1 tsp olive oil

In a small bowl, mash the beans with a spoon until they are smooth. Add the garlic, rosemary, salt and pepper. Heat a non-stick sauté pan, then add oil, swirling it around to coat the pan. Add bean mixture, and cook over medium heat for 5 minutes or until hot.

Spread one-third of the bean mixture onto a tortilla. Roll the tortilla jelly-roll fashion. Repeat with the rest of the mixture and the remaining tortillas. Cut each roll-up in five pieces and serve immediately.

The roll-ups can be wrapped in foil and kept warm in a 225° oven until ready to serve.

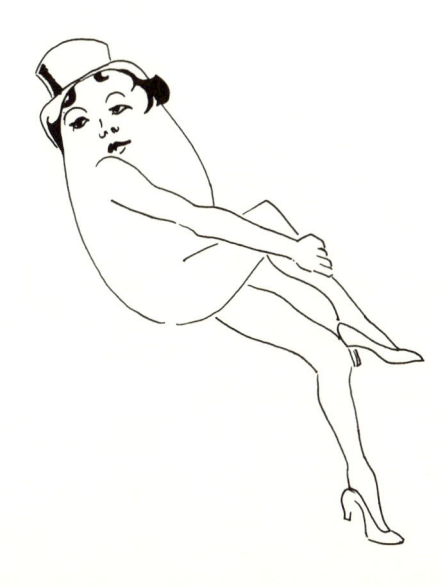

Eggplant Dip

Makes 2¼ cups
2 grams per ¼ cup

1 large eggplant
1 medium onion, diced
3 Tbs lemon juice
1 Tbs olive oil
1 tsp sugar
2-3 garlic cloves, pressed or minced
¼-½ tsp salt

Preheat oven to 450°. Prick the eggplant with a fork in several places. Put the eggplant on a baking sheet and bake for 40 minutes, until the skin turns dark brown.

Cool the eggplant until it can be handled. Peel off skin with your fingers. Cut the eggplant into chunks and put in a blender or food processor. Add the remaining ingredients and process until smooth. Check seasoning. Chill for 1 hour before serving.

Serve with herbed crostini, pita triangles, crackers or crudités.

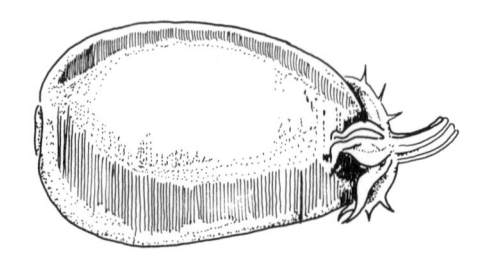

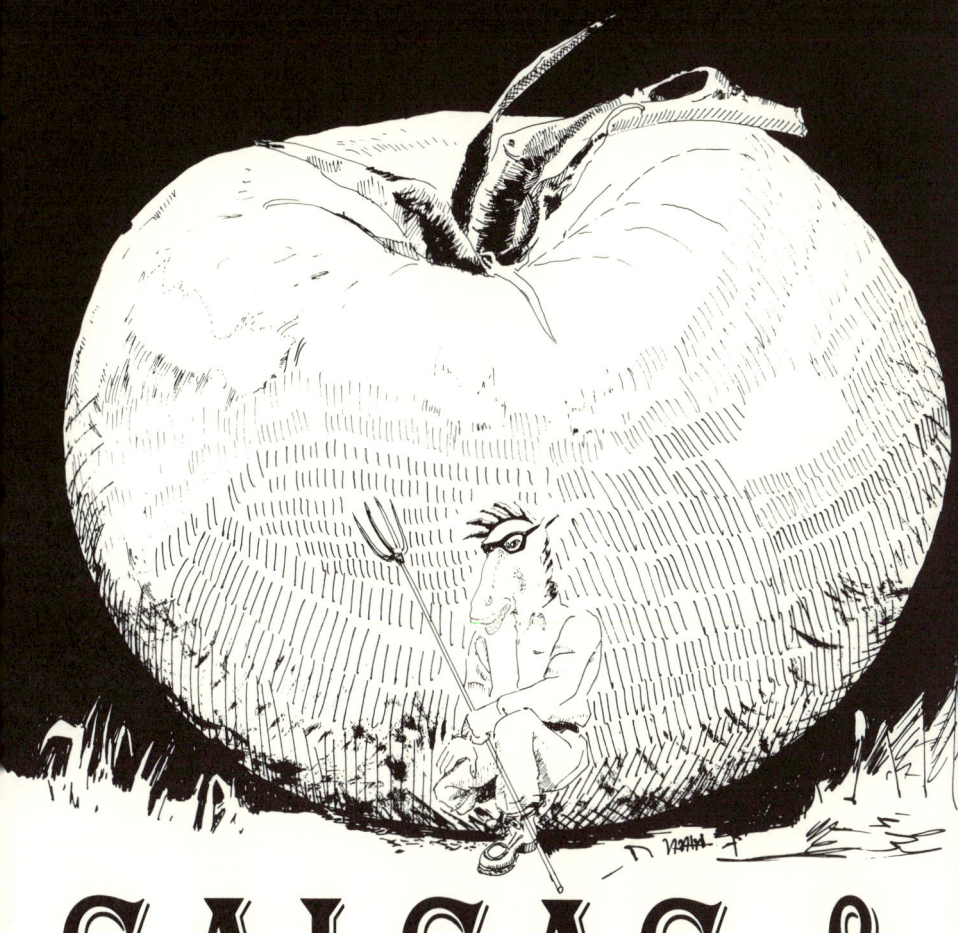

SALSAS & COMPANY

Mango Salsa

Makes 2½ cups
0 grams per ¼ cup

Use your favorite brand of bottled salsa to make this quick and easy salsa.

    1 large ripe mango
    1¼ cups tomato-based salsa
    2 scallions, chopped
    ¼ cup cilantro, minced
    1 Tbs fresh lime juice

Peel, pit, and coarsely dice the mango. In a medium serving bowl, add the mango and the remaining ingredients, stirring well. Serve cold.

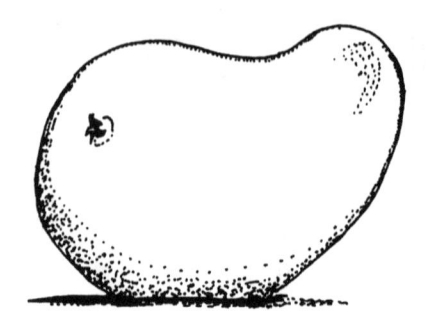

Salsa Verde

Makes 2 cups
0 grams per ¼ cup

Great on grilled fish or chicken. Or use as a chip dip. The salsa will keep several days in the refrigerator.

3 Anaheim peppers
1 lb (about 12) fresh tomatillos, husked
1 clove garlic
¼ cup fresh cilantro leaves
1 jalapeño, seeded
½ cup water
1 tsp salt
1 medium onion, chopped

Roast the peppers on a grill or under a broiler until lightly charred all over. Place the peppers in a paper bag to steam them and facilitate removal of the skins. When cool, remove the skins, stems and seeds.

Place the tomatillos in a medium saucepan and cover with water. Over medium heat, cook the tomatillos until they are soft, about 10 minutes.

In a food processor or blender, mince the garlic, cilantro and jalapeño pepper. Add the tomatillos, roasted Anaheim peppers, water and salt, to the food processor or blender, blending until smooth. Transfer to a bowl and stir in the chopped onions. Chill in the refrigerator for at least 1 hour before serving.

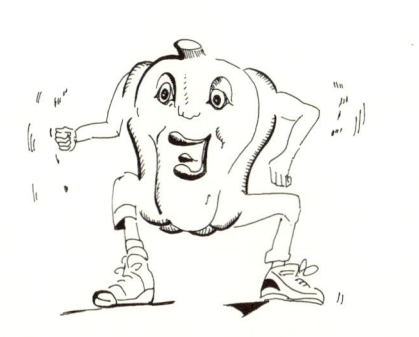

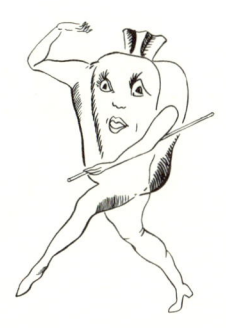

Apple Butter

Makes 2 cups
0 grams per ¼ cup

A great afternoon snack when spread on graham crackers, or on rice cakes, and topped with a sliced banana.

    2 lbs. ripe apples
    ½ cup apple cider
    ¾ cup brown sugar, firmly packed
    1 Tbs cinnamon
    ¼ tsp allspice
    ¼ tsp ground cloves

Peel, core, and slice the apples. Place apples and the cider in a medium saucepan and cook until tender, about 10 minutes. Stir in the spices and cook 5 minutes more, stirring frequently to keep mixture from sticking. When the butter is cool, puree in a food processor or blender. Spoon the mixture into clean jars and refrigerate for up to 4-6 weeks. Can be frozen in plastic containers for up to nine months.

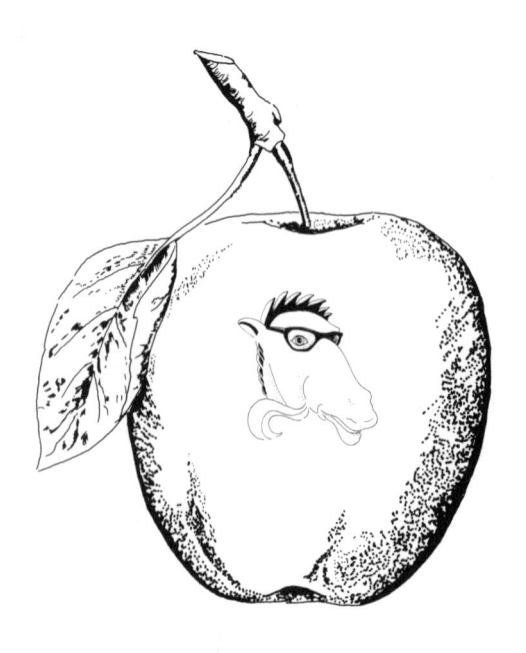

Devil's Sauce

Makes 1¼ cups
1 gram per ¼ cup

In Zeb's household, a standing rib roast is always served on Christmas Day. The next day, Boxing Day, this sauce (adapted from a James Beard recipe) is served over the sliced beef leftovers.

    2 10-oz cans beef broth, skimmed of fat
    1 tsp butter
    3 shallots, finely minced
    1 Tbs Worcestershire sauce
    juice of 1 lemon
    Tabasco
    1 Tbs Dijon-style mustard
    1 Tbs flour

In a medium saucepan heat the beef broth and reduce to 1 cup. Add the butter, shallots, Worcestershire sauce, lemon, Tabasco, and mustard. Stir well until heated through. A few minutes before serving, thicken the sauce by slowly whisking in the flour.

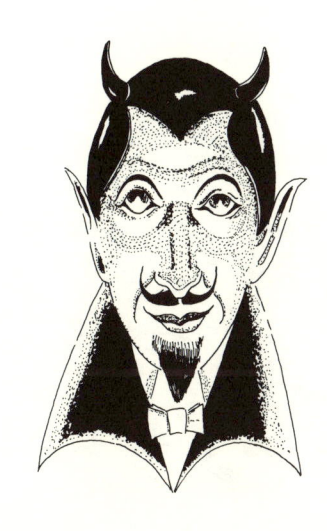

Bread and Butter Pickles

Makes 2 quarts
0 grams per ½ cup

Take advantage of summer's bountiful cucumber crop. Select only the freshest, smallest, unwaxed pickling cucumbers—about five pounds—and let the food processor's slicing blade make short work of the slicing. The pickles will keep for a year without spoiling in the refrigerator—if they last that long.

    10 cups unpeeled pickling cucumbers, sliced
    1 sweet red pepper, chopped
    1 cup fresh or frozen pearl onions (defrost, if frozen)
    2 cups sugar
    1 cup cider vinegar
    2 Tbs kosher salt
    1 Tbs each: celery seed, mustard seed, dill weed

Pack half the sliced cucumbers, half the red pepper and a half cup onions into each of two 1-quart jars. In a large mixing bowl, stir together the sugar, vinegar, salt, celery seed, mustard seed and dill weed until the sugar and spice are well blended.

Pour the liquid into the quart jars, filling almost to the brim. Cover and refrigerate for 4 weeks before using.

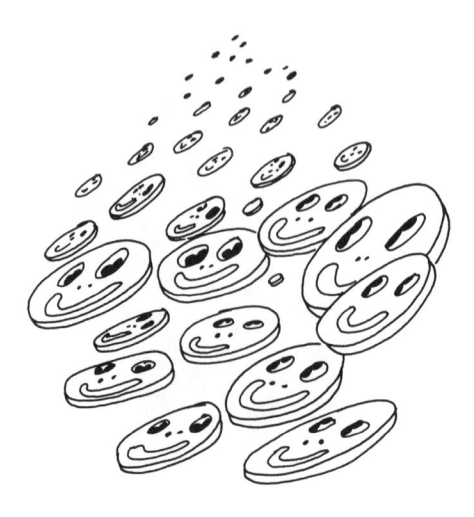

Quick Raisin Sauce

Makes 2 cups
0 grams per ¼ cup

Leftover turkey or chicken? A quick, no-fat sauce packed with flavor.

- ½ cup raisins
- ½ cup cider vinegar
- ½ cup brown sugar
- 1-2 Tbs Dijon-style mustard
- ¼ tsp salt
- 1 Tbs cornstarch

Plump the raisins in a glass of water for ten minutes.

Place 1 ½ cups water into a medium saucepan; bring to a boil. Stir in the vinegar, brown sugar, mustard and salt. Whisk in the cornstarch and stir on high heat until thick. Drain the water from the raisins and add to the sauce. Heat through on medium-low heat.

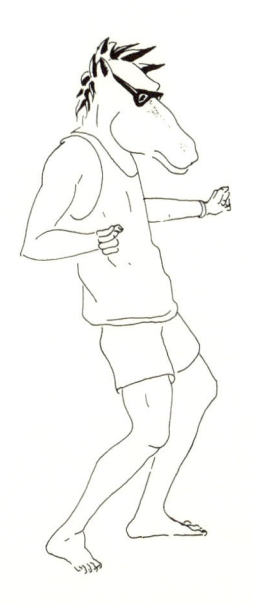

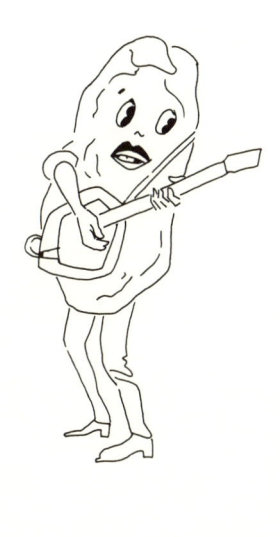

No-Cook Chutney

Serves 4
0 grams per serving

4 tart apples, washed and cored
3 stalks celery
¼ cup finely-chopped onion
½ cup raisins
2 Tbs lemon juice
¼ tsp each: Allspice and cayenne pepper
2 tsp grated ginger (powdered may be substituted)
salt, to taste

Chop apples and celery into bite-size chunks.

Blend all ingredients in a mixing bowl. Check seasonings, adding more if necessary. Cover and refrigerate. Will keep for 1 week.

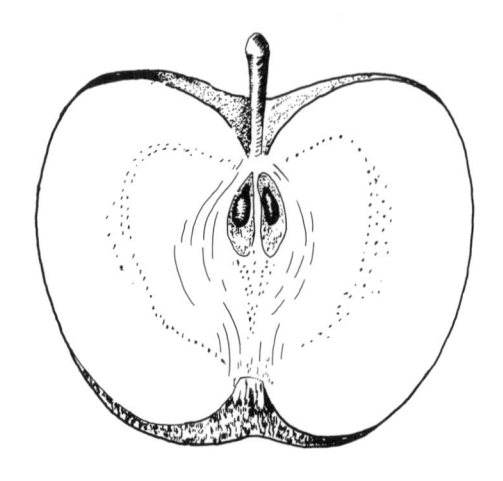

Apricot Chutney

Makes approx. 1 quart
0 grams per serving

Chutney is a versatile condiment to have in your fridge. Spoon it over meat, cover and bake, and it will naturally tenderize any cut. Mix with cream cheese and it becomes a tantalizing dip for crudités. Purchased chutney is very expensive in proportion to the quantity sold in those meager glass bottles. Chutney can be assembled in 10 minutes and half an hour later you have a quart of valuable chutney. Chutney made from dried apricots is particularly convenient because dried apricots save the work of peeling and coring fruit. Try to buy sulfite-free dried apricots, available at health food stores.

- 2 cups dried apricots, washed and sliced
- 2 Tbs fresh ginger, minced
- 1 cup golden seedless raisins
- 1 cup onions, chopped
- 1 lemon, seeded and chopped
- 2 cups brown sugar
- 1 cup cider vinegar
- 2 garlic cloves, minced
- 1½ tsp dry mustard
- 1 jalapeño, seeded and diced
- ½ tsp each: cinnamon, cloves, allspice
- 1 tsp salt

Blend all ingredients in a heavy saucepan and simmer over low heat for approximately 30 minutes.

When cool, place in clean jars. Further processing is not necessary if the chutney is refrigerated.

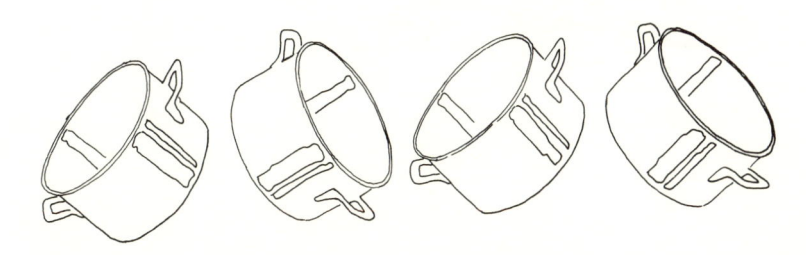

Pineapple Salsa

Makes about 3 cups
0 grams per ¼ cup

Cool, crisp, and colorful, pineapple salsa is a worthy accompaniment to grilled fish or fowl—or spoon some into a bean burrito for something different.

    3 cups fresh pineapple, cored and diced
    ½ cup red pepper, diced
    2 green onions, chopped
    1 jalapeño or serrano chili, minced
    2 tsp fresh mint or cilantro, chopped
    1 Tbs fresh lime juice

Combine ingredients in a large bowl. Refrigerate for at least 1 hour before serving. Will keep, refrigerated, for up to 3 days.

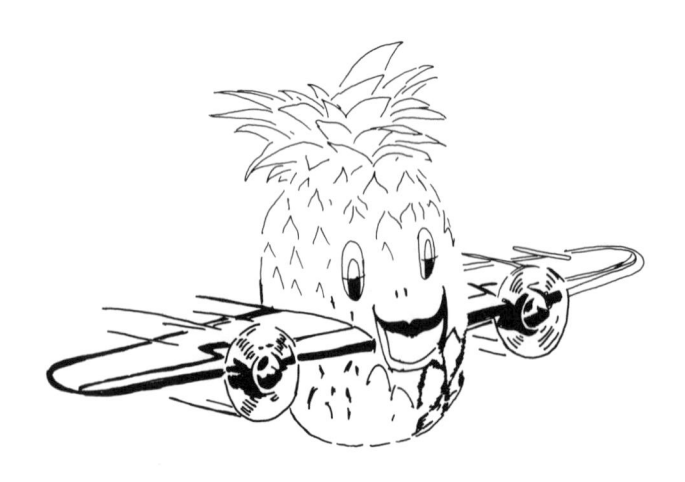

Corn Relish

Makes 2 cups
0 grams per ¼ cup

Corn relish, one of those old-fashioned condiments, is a fat-watcher's pal. Serve it on the side with tuna or turkey burgers. A fresh batch makes a welcome gift.

¼ cup cider vinegar
¼ cup water
¼ cup sugar
1 Tbs cornstarch
1 tsp turmeric
½ tsp celery seeds
2 Tbs onion, minced
1 10-oz package frozen corn, thawed
2 Tbs green pepper, chopped
2 Tbs red pepper or pimento, diced
salt, to taste

In a medium saucepan, combine the cider vinegar, water, sugar, cornstarch, turmeric and celery seeds, stirring until smooth. Add the onion. Cook over medium heat, stirring constantly until mixture boils, then boil for 1 minute more.

Remove from heat. Stir in corn, green and red pepper (or pimento). Season with salt, to taste. Place in a jar and refrigerate until cold.

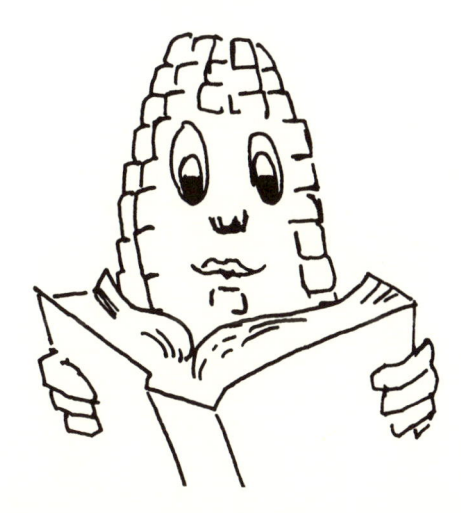

Jalapeño Jelly

Makes 2½ quarts
0 grams per serving

If you've never before tried your hand at making jelly, this could be the recipe for you. Jalapeño jelly is eminently versatile when slathered on corn bread, topping a sweet potato, or dolloped on baked acorn squash. You'll find you don't need that old *minute-on-the-lips-lifetime-on-the-hips butter*. This recipe makes about 10 pints, but it can be halved. One last note—be sure to wear rubber gloves when preparing the chilies.

> 3 cups cider vinegar
> 5 lbs sugar
> 14 jalapeño chilies, seeded and finely minced
> 2 packages (from 1 box) liquid pectin
> 2-3 drops green food color (optional)
> paraffin for sealing jars

In a large saucepan, bring the vinegar and sugar to a boil. Stir until the sugar is dissolved, then reduce heat to medium. Add the chilies and simmer for 10 minutes, skimming foam. Stir in the liquid pectin and return to a boil. Boil for 1 minute. Add the food coloring, if desired. Remove the pan from the heat and let stand for 15 minutes.

Pour into sterilized jars and seal with paraffin. Store in a cool, dark place.

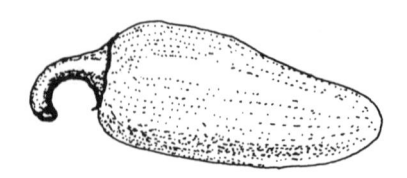

SALADS & DRESSINGS

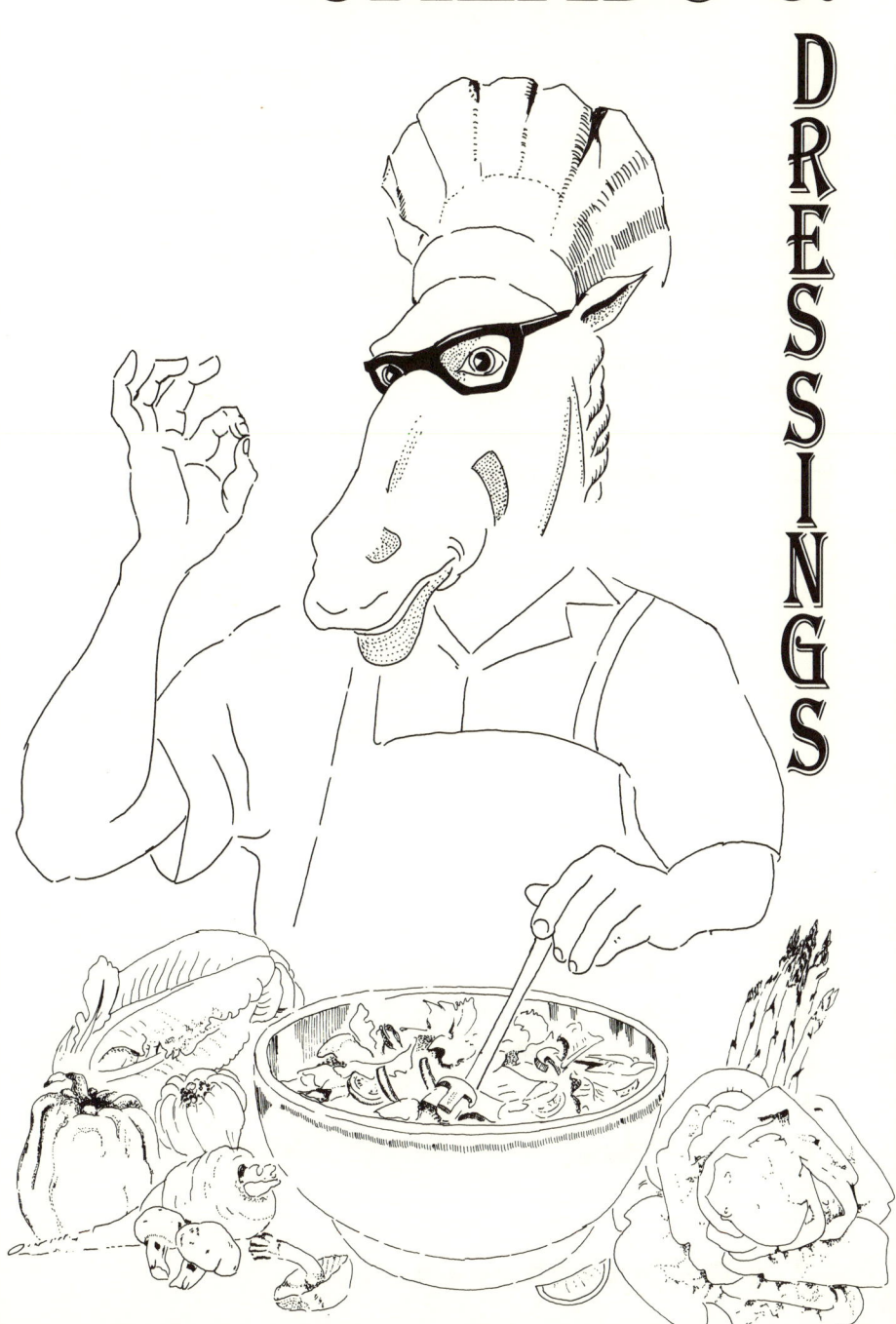

Black Bean Salad

Serves 4
0.5 gram per serving

A salad so tasty, your friends and family will never guess it is prepared without oil.

    1 15-oz can black beans, rinsed and drained
    ½ cup frozen corn kernels
    1 ripe tomato, seeded, peeled and diced
    2 scallions, chopped
    2-3 Tbs fresh minced cilantro
    1-2 garlic cloves, minced
    salt and pepper, to taste
    juice of 1 lime

Put all ingredients except lime juice in a serving bowl. Toss. Squeeze lime juice over salad. Serve very cold.

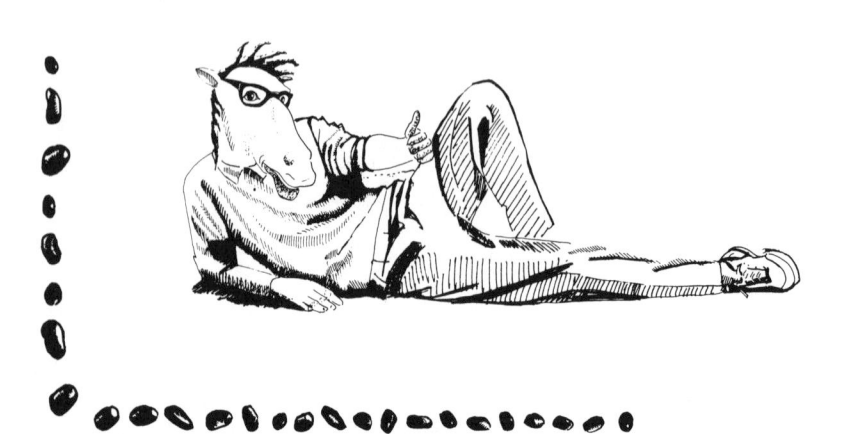

Ruddy Good Slaw

Serves 4
1.2 grams per serving

Purple and orange with a smattering of green, a salad with lots of visual appeal and taste.

    3 cups red cabbage, shredded finely
    3 cups carrots, shredded finely
    ¼ cup scallions, chopped
    ¼ cup apple cider vinegar
    1 tsp oil
    1 Tbs sugar
    ½ tsp salt and pepper

Combine red cabbage, carrots, and scallions into a large bowl. In a small bowl, whisk together vinegar, oil, sugar, salt and pepper. Add to slaw ingredients, stirring well. Cover and refrigerate for 1 hour or more. Before serving, stir again and place in a smaller bowl.

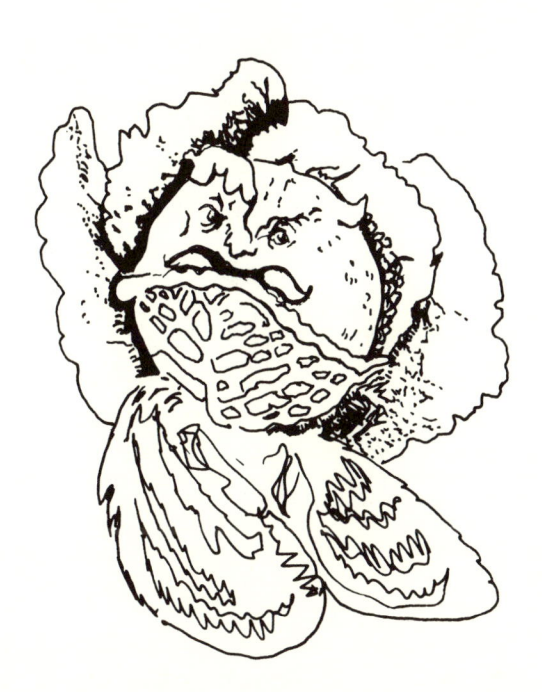

Cucumber Salad

Serves 4
0 grams per serving

2 cucumbers
1 tsp salt
2 Tbs water
2 Tbs malt vinegar
1 Tbs sugar
white pepper, to taste

Wash cucumbers with a drop of detergent to remove as much wax as possible. Slice cucumbers very thinly. Add water and salt and mix well. Cover and refrigerate for 1 hour.

Drain cucumbers and squeeze lightly to get rid of excess water. Add vinegar, sugar and pepper, mixing well.

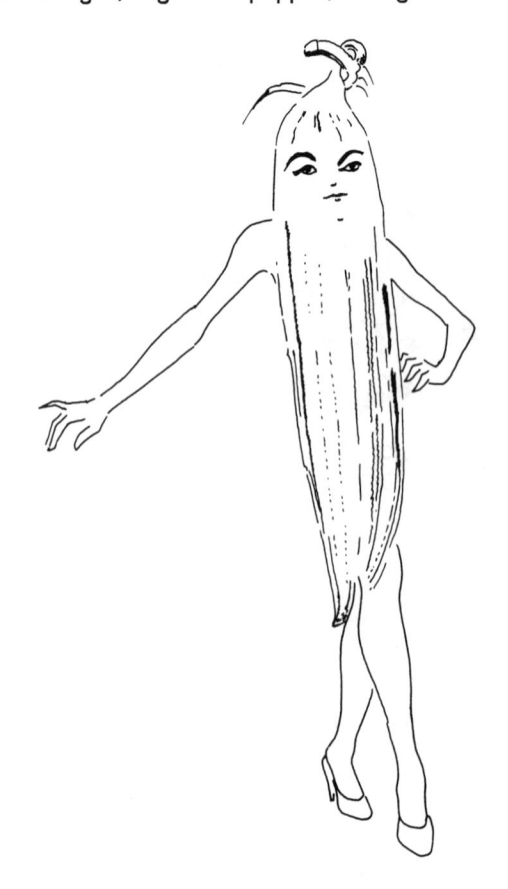

Shredded Carrot Salad

Serves 4
Trace grams per serving

Crushed pineapple adds a sweet tang to this old standby.

    4 large carrots, peeled and grated
    ½ cup raisins
    2 Tbs lemon juice
    2 Tbs honey
    1 8-oz can crushed pineapple, drained

In a medium mixing bowl, add all the ingredients, stirring well. Refrigerate. Prior to serving, stir well again.

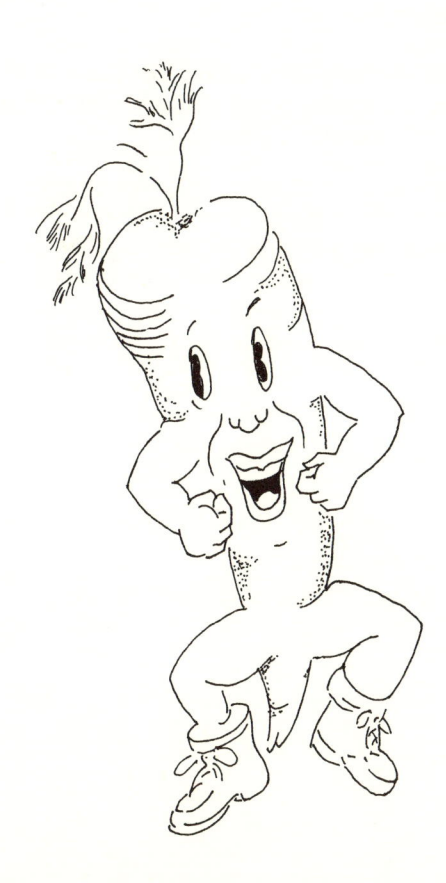

Sauerkraut Salad

Serves 6
0.5 gram per serving

This is a good salad accompaniment for those occasions when the grill is sizzling with low-fat sausages. Prepare the salad the day before for a full blending of flavors.

    4 cups sauerkraut, drained
    ½ cup onions, chopped finely
    ½ cup red pepper, chopped finely
    ½ cup green pepper, chopped finely
    1 cup vinegar
    1 cup sugar

Mix together the sauerkraut, onions, and red and green pepper in a large mixing bowl.

Place the vinegar and sugar in a sauce pan, stir well, and bring to a hard boil. Pour the dressing over the sauerkraut mixture. Place in refrigerator. Will keep for 1 week.

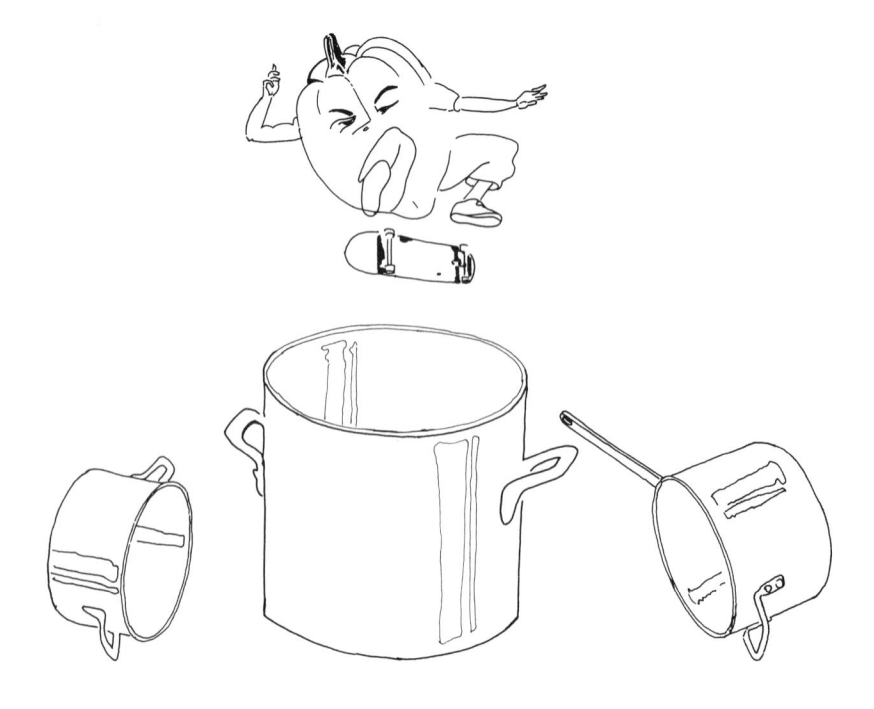

Cherry Tomato Salad

Serves 4
3.5 grams per serving

1 pint cherry tomatoes
¼ cup grated asiago or other hard cheese
1 Tbs red wine vinegar
1 scallion, chopped
1 clove garlic, minced

Rinse cherry tomatoes and remove stems. Cut each cherry tomato in half. Add remaining ingredients. Allow flavors to develop for a couple of hours before serving.

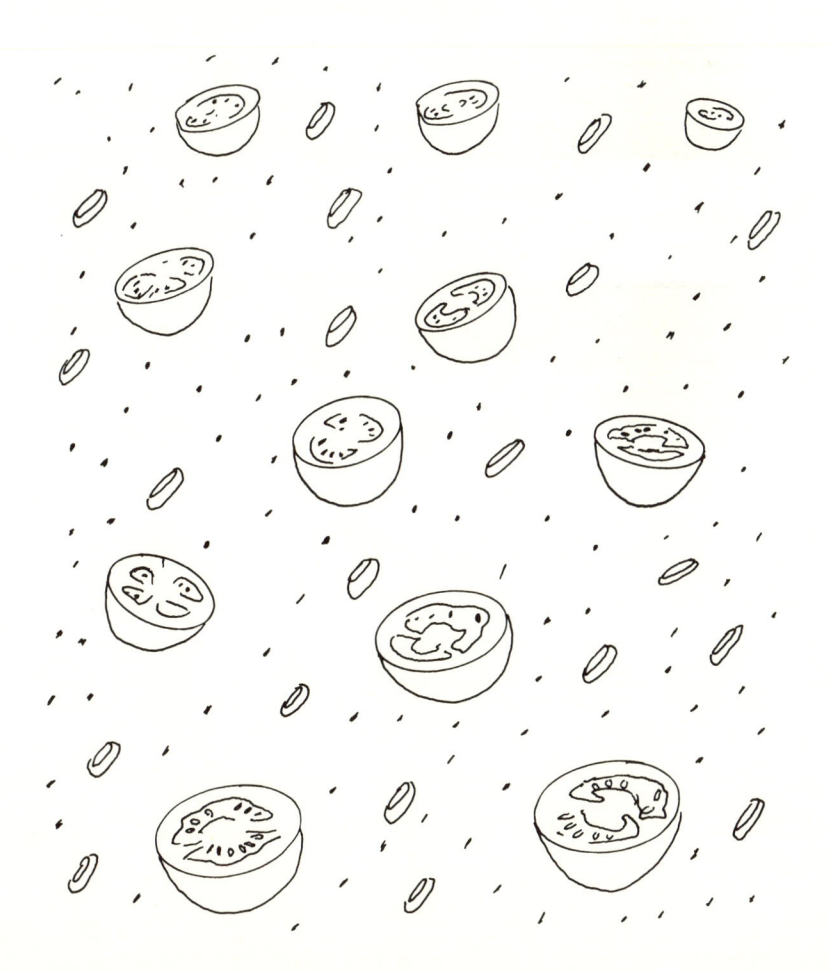

Raita as Salad

Serves 2
0 grams per serving

Raita is well known as a condiment in Indian cuisine. In this version the cucumber is cut into crescent shapes and is served as a salad. This makes a splendid accompaniment to broiled fish or chicken. Recipe can be doubled.

1 cucumber
¼ tsp salt
1 Tbs cumin seeds
2 Tbs cilantro, finely chopped
2 Tbs white onion, finely chopped
2 Tbs nonfat yogurt

Peel cucumber. Cut in half lengthwise. Scoop out the seeds and discard. Slice each cucumber half into ¼" crescents. Place in a small serving bowl and salt the cucumbers.

In a nonstick pan, toast the cumin seeds over medium heat shaking the pan constantly for a couple of minutes. Add cumin, cilantro and onion to the cucumbers. Stir the yogurt into the cucumbers. Cover with plastic wrap, and chill in refrigerator until serving time. Stir raita again before serving.

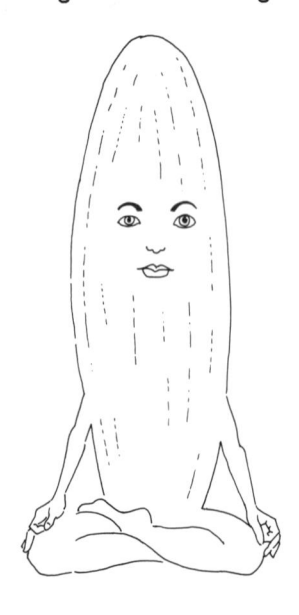

Composed Tomato and Mozzarella Salad

Serves 2
5 grams per serving

Recipe can be doubled or tripled.

    2 plump, juicy summer tomatoes
    2 oz part skim milk mozzarella
    12 fresh basil leaves—chop one for garnish
    good quality red wine vinegar
    salt, to taste, and pepper

Slice tomatoes in ½" rounds. Using a cheese slicer, slice cheese into thin layers, making approximately 20 thin slices of cheese.

In a glass straight-sided bowl, arrange a layer of tomatoes then basil and s&p. Sprinkle over the mixture 1 tsp vinegar. Add a layer of cheese. Repeat the process until all the ingredients are used, ending with a top layer of cheese. Add the chopped basil. To compact the salad, press down lightly with your palms. Refrigerate at least 1 hour.

To serve, cut into pie-shaped wedges.

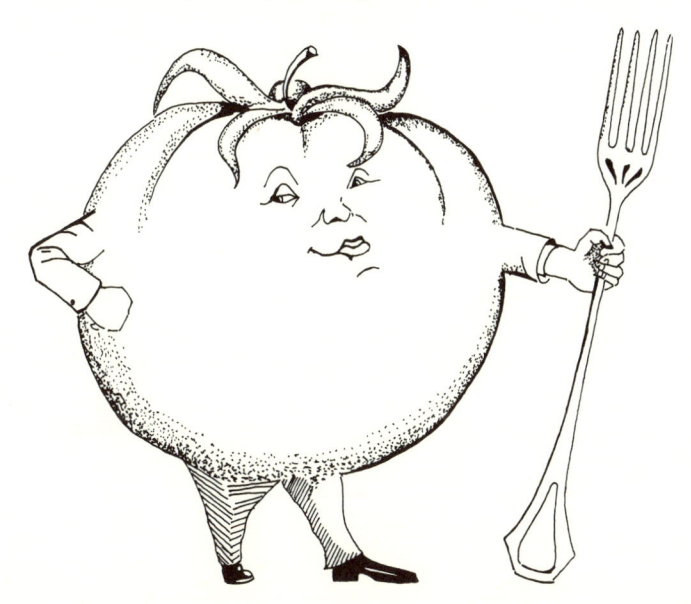

Oriental Dressing (and Marinade)

Serves 2
7.5 grams per serving

An excellent dressing for thinly-sliced cucumber, bean sprouts and shredded carrot with scallion. Double recipe for marinade.

   1 Tbs Oriental sesame oil
   2 Tbs rice vinegar
   1 Tbs low sodium soy sauce
   1 clove garlic, crushed
   ¼ tsp powdered ginger
   dash of Tabasco

Mix all ingredients together in bottom of salad bowl, or place in a cruet and shake.

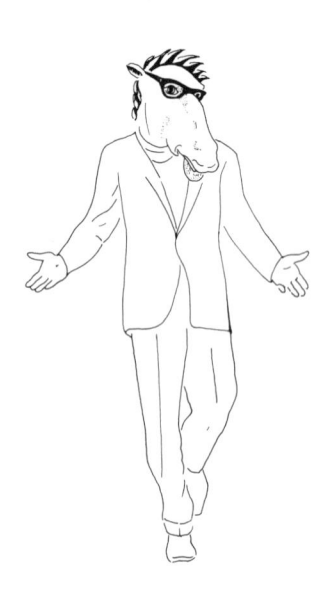

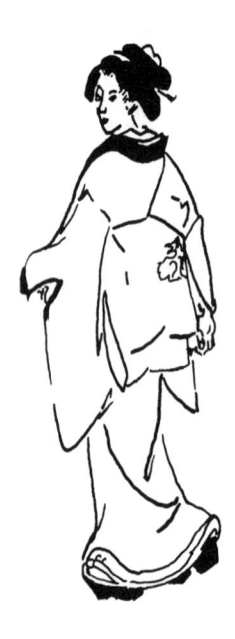

Honey Herb Salad Dressing

Makes approx. 1¼ cups
Trace gram per 2 Tbs

Good on mixed green salads.

¼ cup honey
½ cup tomato juice
2 tsps olive oil
¼ cup red wine vinegar
1 Tbs Worcestershire sauce
1 clove garlic crushed
1 Tbs each: Minced herbs, basil, parsley, oregano
salt, to taste, and pepper

Place ingredients in blender and whir until smooth.

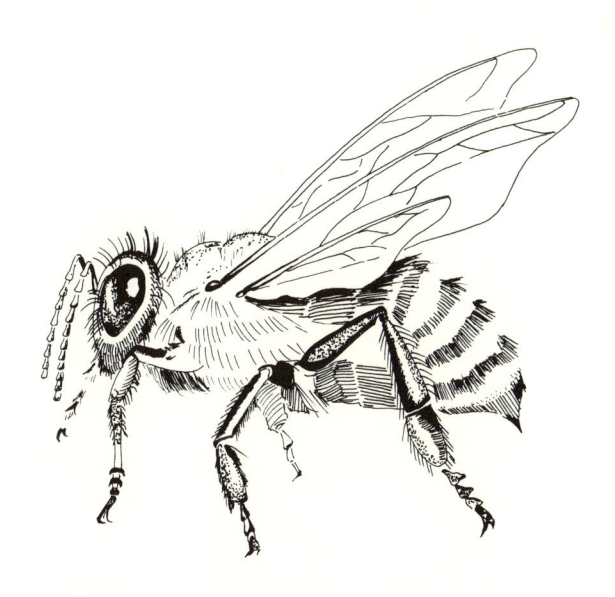

Buttermilk Dressing

Makes approx. 1 ¼ cups
Trace grams per 2 Tbs serving

1 cup buttermilk
1 Tbs Dijon-style mustard
¼ cup grated cucumber
1 chopped green onion
1 Tbs minced parsley or dill
½ tsp salt and pepper, to taste

Whir all ingredients in blender until smooth.

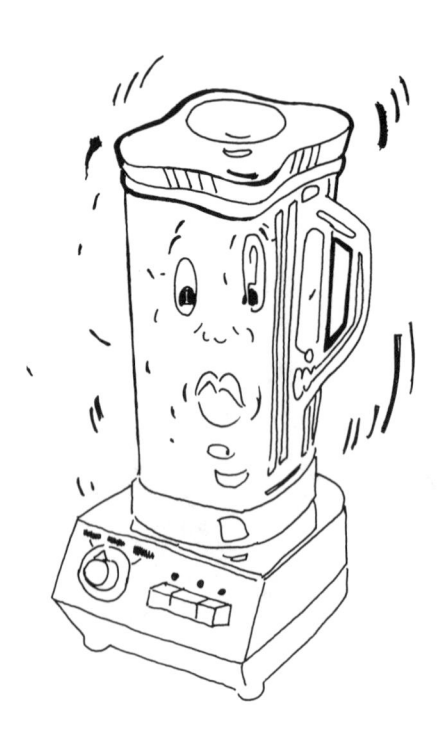

Ranch Dressing

Makes 1 ¼ cups
0 grams per 2 Tbs serving

Best as a summer salad dressing using fresh herbs.

    1 large clove garlic
    1 cup nonfat yogurt
    1 Tbs chives (fresh preferable)
    1 Tbs fresh or dried tarragon
    4-5 fresh basil leaves, or 1 tsp dried
    ¼ tsp celery seed
    ½ tsp onion flakes
    2 tsp Dijon-style mustard
    2 tsp minced fresh parsley
    salt and pepper, to taste
    2 Tbs red wine vinegar

Put garlic in food processor and process until garlic is minced. Add remaining ingredients and pulse until dressing is well blended.

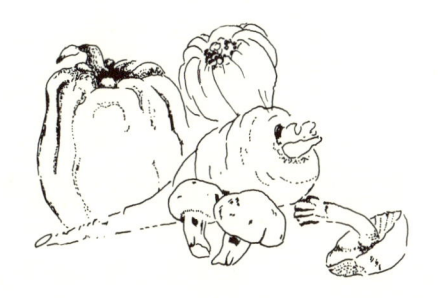

Honey Fruit Salad Dressing

Makes approx. 1 cup
Trace grams per 2 Tbs

A wonderful fruit salad topping, or use it as a dip for fruit. Slice fresh fruit—apples, bananas, kiwi, grapes, oranges—and mingle with berries in season.

    1 cup nonfat yogurt
    3 Tbs honey
    2 Tbs tarragon vinegar or cider vinegar
    1 tsp poppy seeds
    ¼ tsp salt

Place all ingredients in a cruet and shake, or whir in a blender.

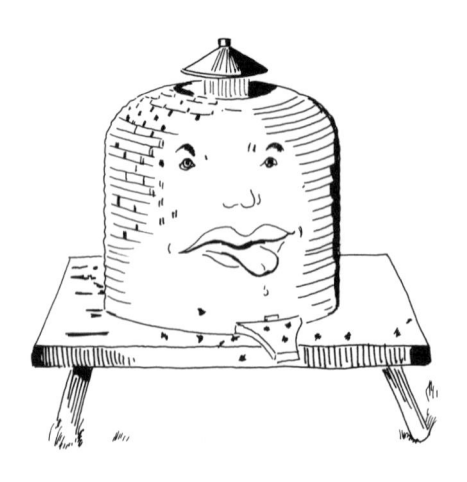

Orange Vinaigrette

Makes ½ cup
0 grams per 2 Tbs

A versatile dressing. Tasty on chef's salad, or try it as a sweet counterpart to watercress.

    juice of 1 orange
    1 Tbs Dijon-style mustard
    2 Tbs honey
    1 clove garlic, crushed
    salt and pepper, to taste

Place all ingredients in a cruet and shake, or whir in a blender.

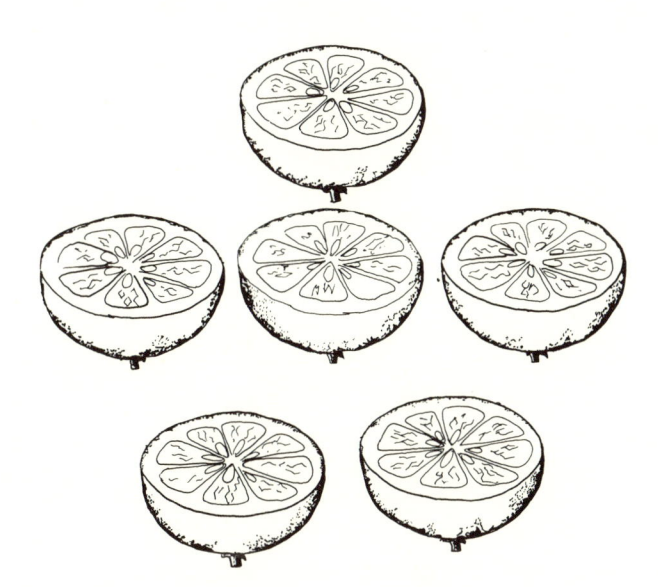

Adults Only Salad Dressing

Makes approx. 2 cups
0 grams per 2 Tbs

An exotic and nippy way to dress your naked greens.

    1 8-oz bottle Pritikin Ranch Dressing (fat- and sodium-free)
    1 14-oz can hearts of palm, chopped
    2 cloves garlic, minced
    3 Tbs capers, drained of liquid
    1 small jar pimentos, diced, or 1 red pepper, diced
    ¼ tsp salt and pepper

Greens: Endive, romaine, bibb, Boston, green onions, etc.

Pour the Ranch dressing into a small sealable bowl. Add the hearts of palm, garlic, capers, and pimentos, or chopped red pepper, salt and pepper and mix until well combined.

Place the greens on individual plates and spoon 2 Tbs dressing over the greens. Keeps well, refrigerated, for 1 week.

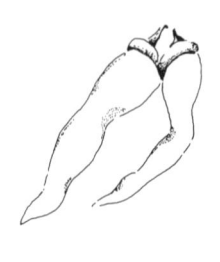

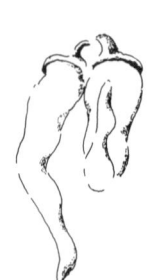

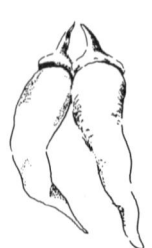

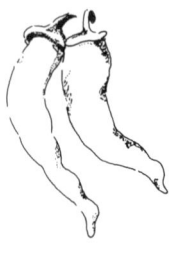

Blue Cheese Dressing

Makes 2 cups
4.1 grams per ¼ cup

For optimum flavor, use the real thing: French Roquefort, Saga Blue, Maytag Blue or Bavarian Blue cheese. To use as a dip, don't thin with milk.

 1 cup fat-free cottage cheese (99%)
 6 Tbs blue cheese, crumbled
 4 Tbs sour half and half
 1 Tbs cider vinegar or lemon juice
 ¼ tsp each, salt and white pepper
 skim milk, to thin dressing if necessary
 1 tsp brandy (optional)

Put cottage cheese, blue cheese, sour half and half, vinegar or lemon juice into a food processor and blend for 10 seconds. Season with salt and pepper. Scrape the sides with a rubber spatula and continue to blend until creamy, adding skim milk a tablespoon at a time until thinned to the desired consistency. Remove from food processor, put in a covered container and stir in brandy, if desired.

Keeps 1 week in the refrigerator in a covered container.

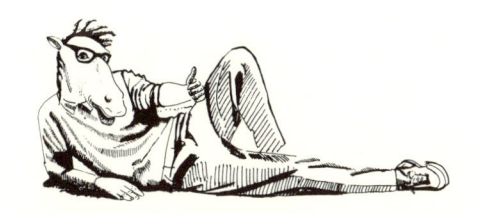

Caesar Dressing

Makes approx. 1 cup
1 gram per ¼ cup

Pour this tangy dressing over romaine lettuce. Toss, then top with croutons and grated cheese. Refrigerate for at least an hour to allow flavors to mingle.

   2 fresh egg whites
   ¼ cup fresh lemon juice
   1 hefty Tbs Dijon-style mustard
   1 tin anchovies
   ¼ cup water
   Tabasco or pepper

Whir the egg whites in a blender, then add the remaining ingredients. Blend until smooth.

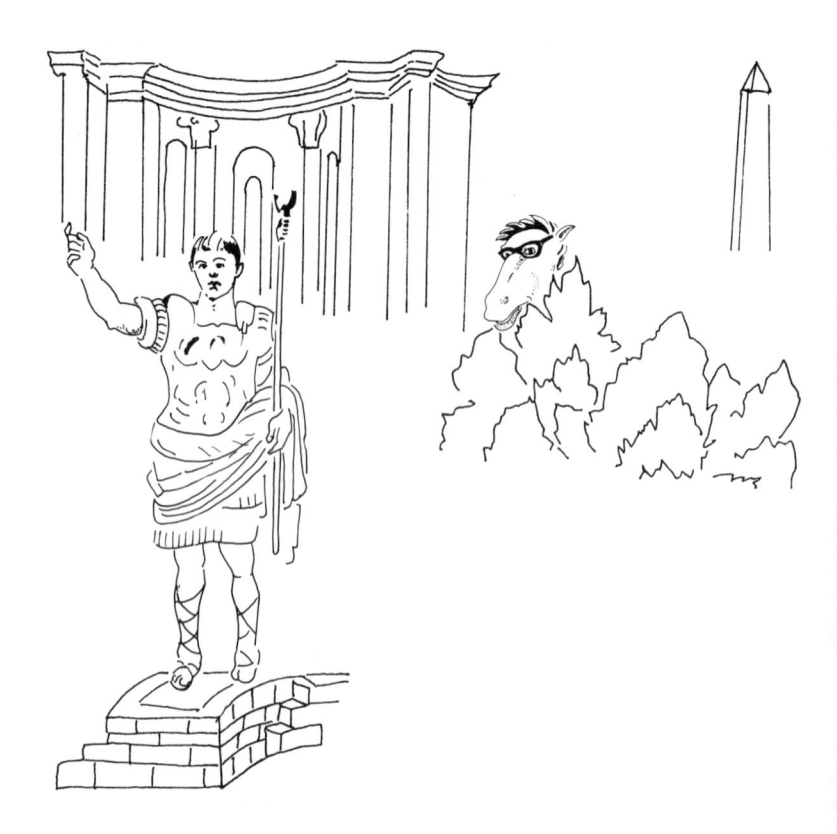

SOUPS

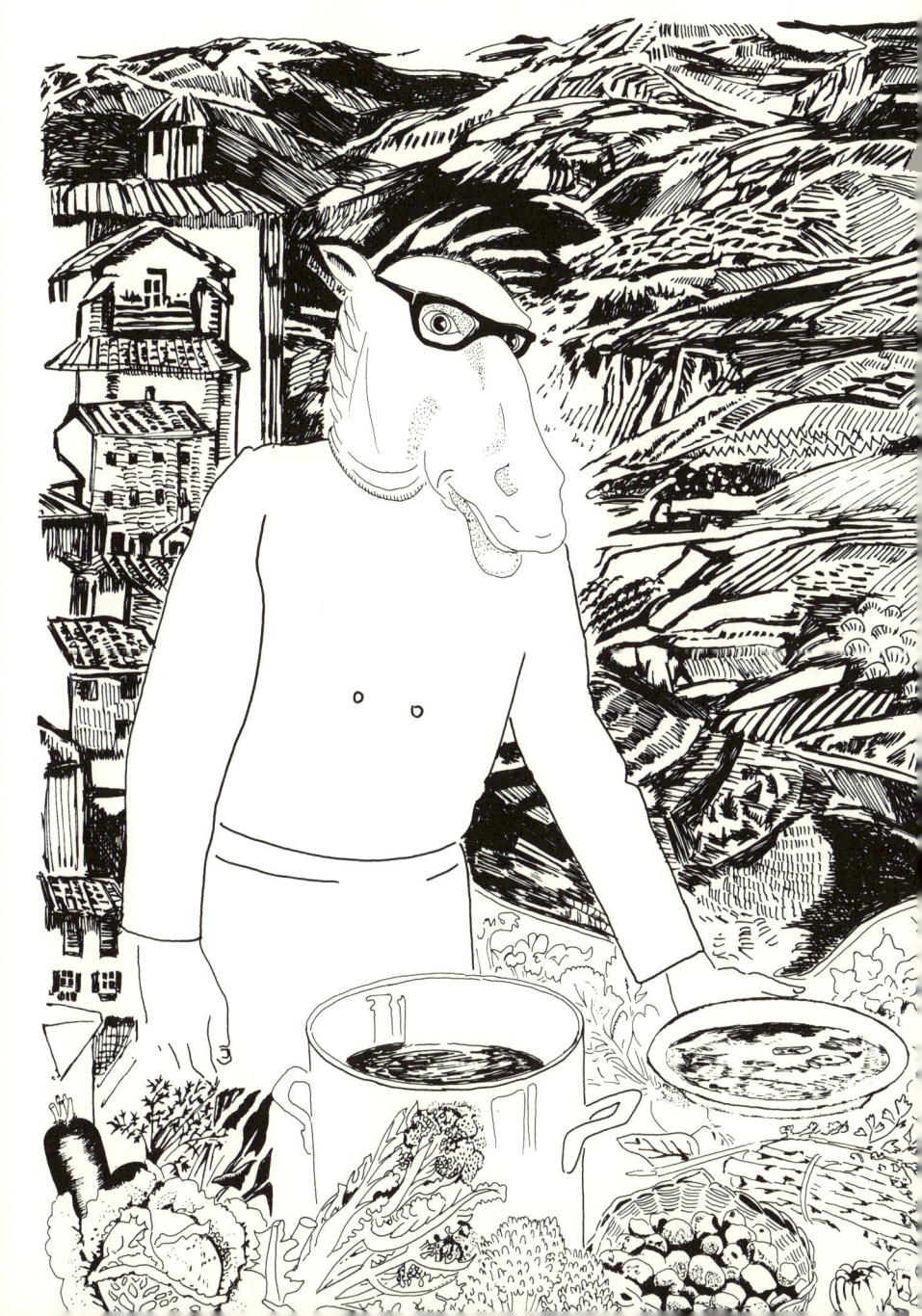

Librada's Cloud Soup

Serves 4
5 grams per serving

This soup always elicits a "Wow!" when the egg white clouds floating on a sea of aromatic broth reach the table.

    3 cups defatted chicken broth
    1 cup nonfat milk
    1 Tbs dry sherry
    ½ tsp salt
    white pepper, to taste
    4 Tbs chopped ham (reserve some for topping)
    4 Tbs chopped shrimp
    3 Tbs scallion, chopped (reserve some for topping)
    6 egg whites

Boil the broth with the milk and sherry in a medium pot. Reduce heat and add salt, pepper, ham, shrimp and scallion.

Using an electric mixer, beat the egg whites until stiff. Add to soup. Cover the soup and steam the whites for 3-4 minutes.

Carefully ladle the soup into serving bowls, topping with the steamed "clouds". Add reserved scallions and ham bits. Serve at once.

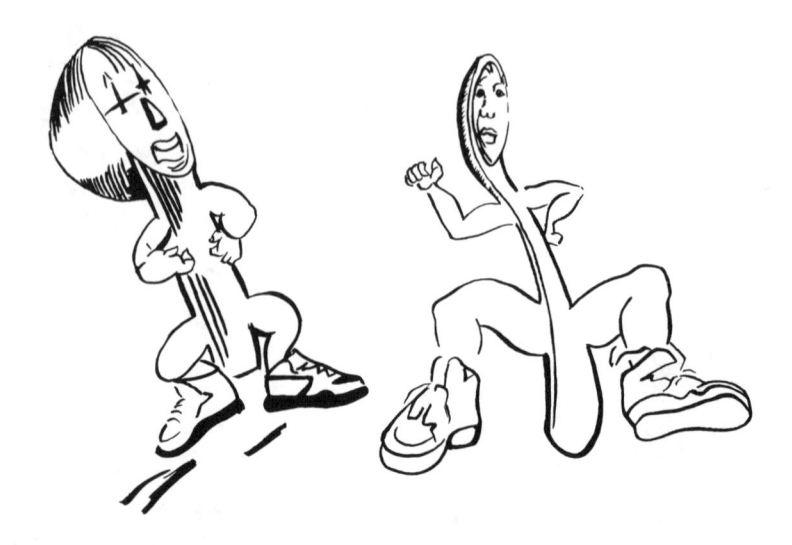

Escarole Soup

Serves 4-6
1.8 grams per serving

A meal in a bowl, and surprisingly easy to make, with less than 2 grams of fat per serving.

- 1 large or 2 small heads escarole lettuce
- 8 cups defatted chicken broth
- ¾ cup small bowtie egg noodles
- 1 clove garlic, minced
- 1 tsp salt
- splash of dry Vermouth (optional)
- fresh ground pepper, to taste
- 4 Tbs grated hard cheese like Parmesan or Asiago

Lop about an inch off the top of the lettuce, discard. Then work your way down to the core, making ½" slices. Discard the core. Wash well to remove the grit. When the lettuce is free of grit, place it in a bowl filled with water, and add 1 tsp salt.

Meanwhile, bring the chicken broth to a boil, then reduce heat to medium-high.

Pour off the water and dry lettuce. Add the lettuce to the broth in batches, stirring frequently. When all the lettuce is incorporated into the broth, simmer for 5 minutes. Add the egg noodles and garlic; stir and cover. Cook the soup on medium heat for about 10 minutes, or until the noodles are done. Taste, add salt, pepper, and Vermouth, if desired. Ladle into warmed soup bowls and top with equal portions of grated cheese.

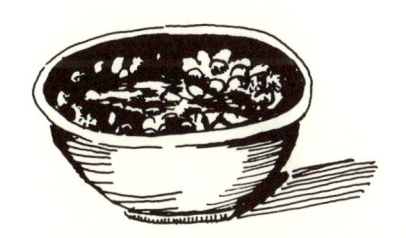

One-Two-Three Soup

Serves 4
1.5 grams per serving

Zeb's grandmère, who was bred in Alsace-Lorraine made this soup for her brood from vegetables in the root cellar when there was precious little else to eat.

- 1 large parsnip, peeled
- 2 large carrots, peeled
- 3 large potatoes, peeled
- 3 Tbs fresh parsley, minced
- salt, to taste and pepper
- 4 Tbs sour half & half

Cut parsnip, carrots, and potatoes into match sticks, or shred with the shredder blade of a food processor. Place vegetables in a medium pot with salt and add 4 cups water. Bring to a boil, then reduce heat and simmer until vegetables are cooked, about 30 minutes.

Add parsley and pepper. Dollop 1 Tbs sour half & half in each of the bowls.

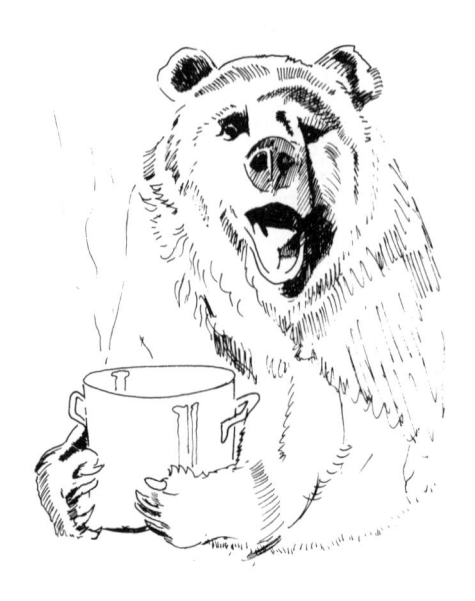

Oriental Chicken Soup

Serves 4
2 grams per serving

A soup that can be prepared in minutes. There is something restorative and comforting about this soup—particularly good to help chase away a cold. The soup can also be made with roast pork: Use pork-flavored Ramen noodles with leftover pork roast, or purchase from the deli counter ¼ pound thinly-sliced roast pork. Cut the pork into bite-size strips.

> 2 10-oz cans chicken broth
> 2 packages chicken-flavored Ramen noodles
> ¼ lb. mushrooms, sliced
> 1 3.5-oz chicken breast, cooked
> ¼ lb. pea pods, or ¼ cup green peas
> 1 tsp soy sauce, or to taste
> 1 scallion, sliced thinly
> ¼ tsp ground ginger (optional)
> 1 small can water chestnuts (optional)

In a 2-quart sauce pan, bring to a boil the chicken broth and the contents of the chicken-flavored packets. (Omit if on a sodium-restricted diet.) Add mushrooms, and simmer until just cooked. Cut the chicken into bite-size strips and add to the broth. Add noodles, and cook for 3 minutes or according to package instructions. Add remaining ingredients and heat through. Serve at once.

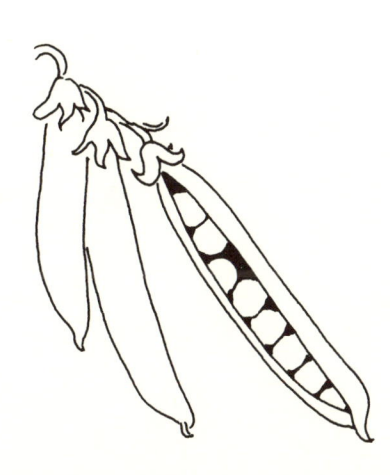

Macaroni, Bean and Spinach Soup

Serves 4
3.7 grams per serving

A robust soup in a clear broth, with fresh spinach and the tang of lemon. With canned cannellini beans, this soup can be prepared very quickly.

- ¾ cup elbow macaroni
- 4 cups beef broth
- 3 cloves garlic, minced
- 2 tsp salt
- 1 tsp crumbled rosemary
- 1 16-oz canned cannellini beans
- 1 Tbs olive oil
- white pepper, to taste
- 10-oz fresh spinach, washed and chopped
- juice of 1 lemon

Cook the pasta according to package directions.

To kettle, add beef broth, garlic, salt, rosemary and beans. Bring to a boil, then reduce heat to low. Stir in the cooked pasta, olive oil and white pepper. One minute before serving, add the spinach and lemon juice.

Serve at once.

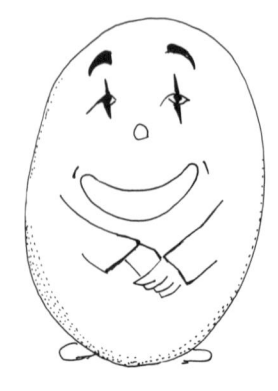

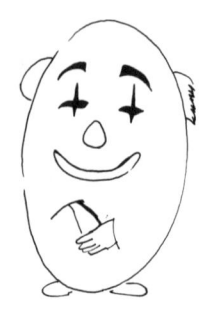

Pepper Cream Soup

Serves 4-6
0 grams per serving

A Tuscan delight without a drop of cream.

    4 sweet red peppers
    1 medium potato
    1 medium onion
    6 cups defatted chicken broth
    ¼ tsp thyme
    1 clove
    2 bay leaves
    salt and pepper, to taste

Remove stem and seeds from peppers. Chop peppers into small pieces. Peel and chop potatoes, and dice the onion.

Put the broth in a large soup kettle and bring to a boil. Tie a cheesecloth bag with thyme, clove and bay leaves, adding it to the soup pot, along with the peppers, onion and potato. Reduce heat to moderate. Cook for 1 hour or until vegetables are very soft.

Remove the cheesecloth bag. Put 2 cups of the soup in a blender and whir until smooth. Put the pureed soup in a large mixing bowl, repeating the process until all the soup is blended. Pour the soup from the mixing bowl back into the kettle and warm through.

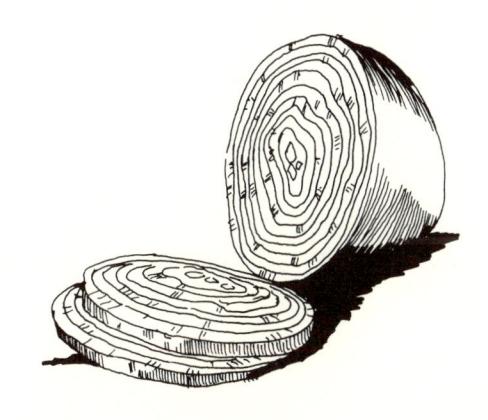

Black Bean Soup with Shrimp

Serves 8
2.4 grams per serving

This soup makes a grand presentation: The velvety black bean background, topped with sour half & half, dotted with green onion and pink shrimp becomes a gustatory picture. If time is a restriction, canned broth is a good substitute for homemade stock. And, instead of soaking the beans, use 2 15-oz cans black beans.

2 ham hocks	¼ cup dry sherry
1 onion, chopped	2 cups dried black beans
2 ribs celery, chopped	1 14½-oz can stewed tomatoes
1 carrot, chopped	
2 cloves garlic	½ lb. cooked shrimp
1 tsp each: dried oregano, basil, thyme and cumin	sour half and half
	2 scallions, chopped
4-5 peppercorns	

Boil 10 cups water in a stock pot. Add the ham hocks and reduce heat. Add the onion, celery, carrot, 1 clove minced garlic, and oregano, basil, thyme and peppercorns. Simmer for 2-3 hours. With a cheesecloth-lined sieve, strain the stock and skim off the fat. (If time permits, refrigerate the stock until the fat hardens.) Reserve the meat from the ham hocks for another use. There should be 8 cups of stock.

Put the strained stock in the stock pot. Add the beans to the stock pot. (If using canned beans, do not drain.) Add the stewed tomatoes, cumin, and 1 remaining clove garlic. Cook the beans until thoroughly cooked, about 2-3 hours.

10 minutes before serving, add the shrimp and sherry. Ladle the soup into bowls, add the chopped scallion and dollop 1 tablespoon sour half & half into each bowl.

Note: If using canned broth, put 4 cups canned chicken and/or vegetable broth into a stock pot with 4 cups water, and bring to a boil. Add onion, carrot, celery, 1 clove garlic, and oregano, basil, thyme and peppercorns. Cook until the vegetables are soft. Strain the stock.

Velvet Summer Squash Soup

Serves 4
0 grams per serving

When all the elements fit: Summer's peak squash, and a leftover baked sweet potato from the night before will result in an easy delight.

- 4-5 summer (yellow) squash, sliced in 1" disks
- 1 14.5-oz can chicken broth (or homemade)
- 1 cooked sweet potato
- ¼ tsp powdered ginger
- ¼ tsp white pepper
- salt, to taste

Place squash and chicken broth in a medium sauce pot. Add water to barely cover squash.

Bring to a boil, then lower heat and simmer on low heat for 15 minutes or until squash is fork tender. Mash sweet potato with a fork and stir into pot. Add powdered ginger, white pepper and salt.

Place mixture in a blender and whir until smooth. Pour back in sauce pan and keep warm until serving time or refrigerate and serve cold.

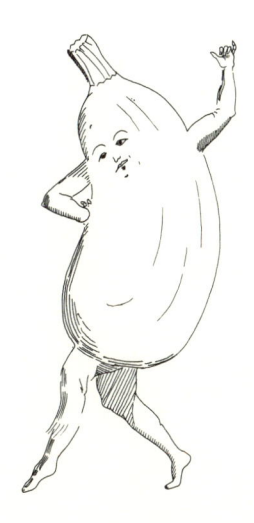

Laurie Colwin's Curried Broccoli Soup

Serves 4
0 grams per serving

A hearty soup with lots of attitude but no fat. It was created by the late Laurie Colwin, a fine writer and inspired cook.

  5 cups chicken broth
  1 large head broccoli, chopped
  1 medium potato, peeled and diced
  2 garlic cloves, minced
  1 tsp curry powder (or more)
  salt and pepper, to taste
  ½-¾ cup nonfat yogurt

Bring the chicken broth to a boil in a soup kettle. Add the broccoli, potato, garlic, curry powder, salt and pepper. Simmer the soup for 20 minutes, or until the vegetables are very tender.

Ladle the vegetables into a blender with about a cup of the stock. Add the yogurt to taste and whir the soup into a purée. Return the puréed soup to the kettle and reheat.

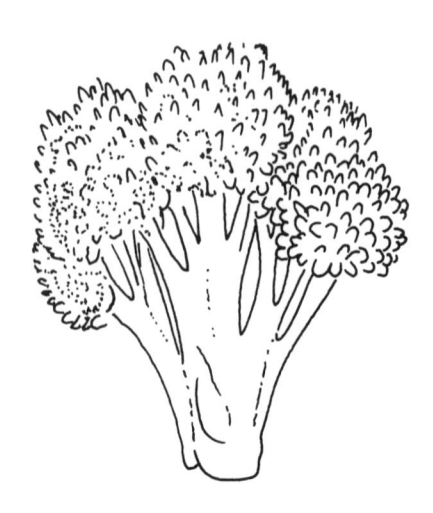

Greek Lemon Soup

Serves 4
2.5 grams per serving

Yummy. A comforting soup. Try adding a bunch of chopped watercress to the soup before incorporating the egg-lemon mixture.

    6 cups defatted chicken broth
    1/3 cup white rice
    1/4 cup lemon juice
    2 egg yolks
    1 bunch watercress, chopped, if desired

Bring stock to a boil in a soup kettle.

Add rice slowly to the boiling chicken stock and cook for 30 minutes until it is very soft. Beat the yolks thoroughly with the lemon juice in a 2-cup bowl. Slowly stir 1 cup hot chicken stock to the egg and lemon mixture, then stir rapidly once it is combined.

(If preparing soup with watercress, add it now.) Remove the broth from the heat and when it has stopped boiling, stir in the egg-broth mixture. Stir rapidly to prevent the soup from curdling. Serve immediately.

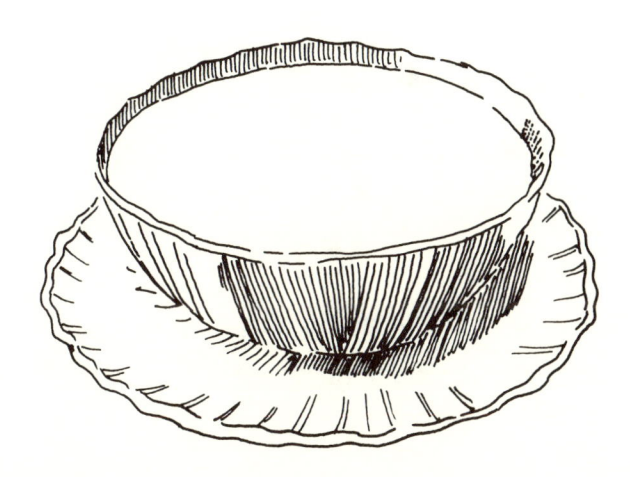

Lentil & Brown Rice Soup

Serves 4-6
0 grams per serving

Feeling virtuous...Want to? Then this is the soup for you.

¾ cup lentils
½ cup raw brown rice
6 cups water
1 Tbs soy sauce or tamari
½ tsp ground cumin
fresh ground pepper, to taste
1 1.5-oz packet onion soup mix
Either: 1 stalk broccoli, diced, ½ cup grated carrot, *or* 1 cup spinach cut in ½" strips
2 Tbs chopped cilantro or parsley
3 Tbs lemon juice

Put lentils, rice, water, soy sauce, cumin, pepper and onion soup mix in a 4-quart pot. Heat to boiling, then cover and simmer, stirring occasionally for about 40 minutes, or until rice and lentils are tender.

Stir in your choice of broccoli, carrot or spinach. Add cilantro and lemon juice and heat until veggies are cooked. Serve with additional cilantro and a lemon slice, if desired.

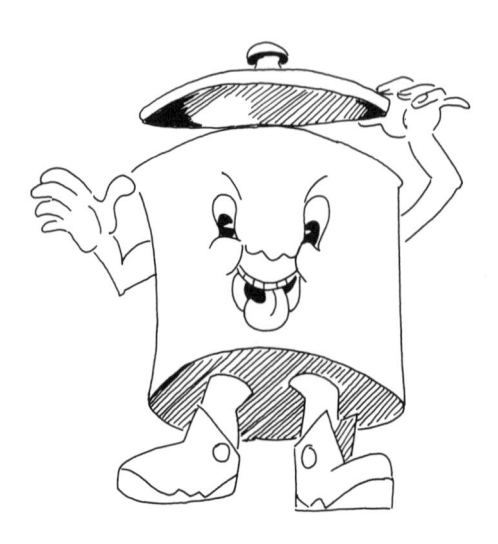

PASTA

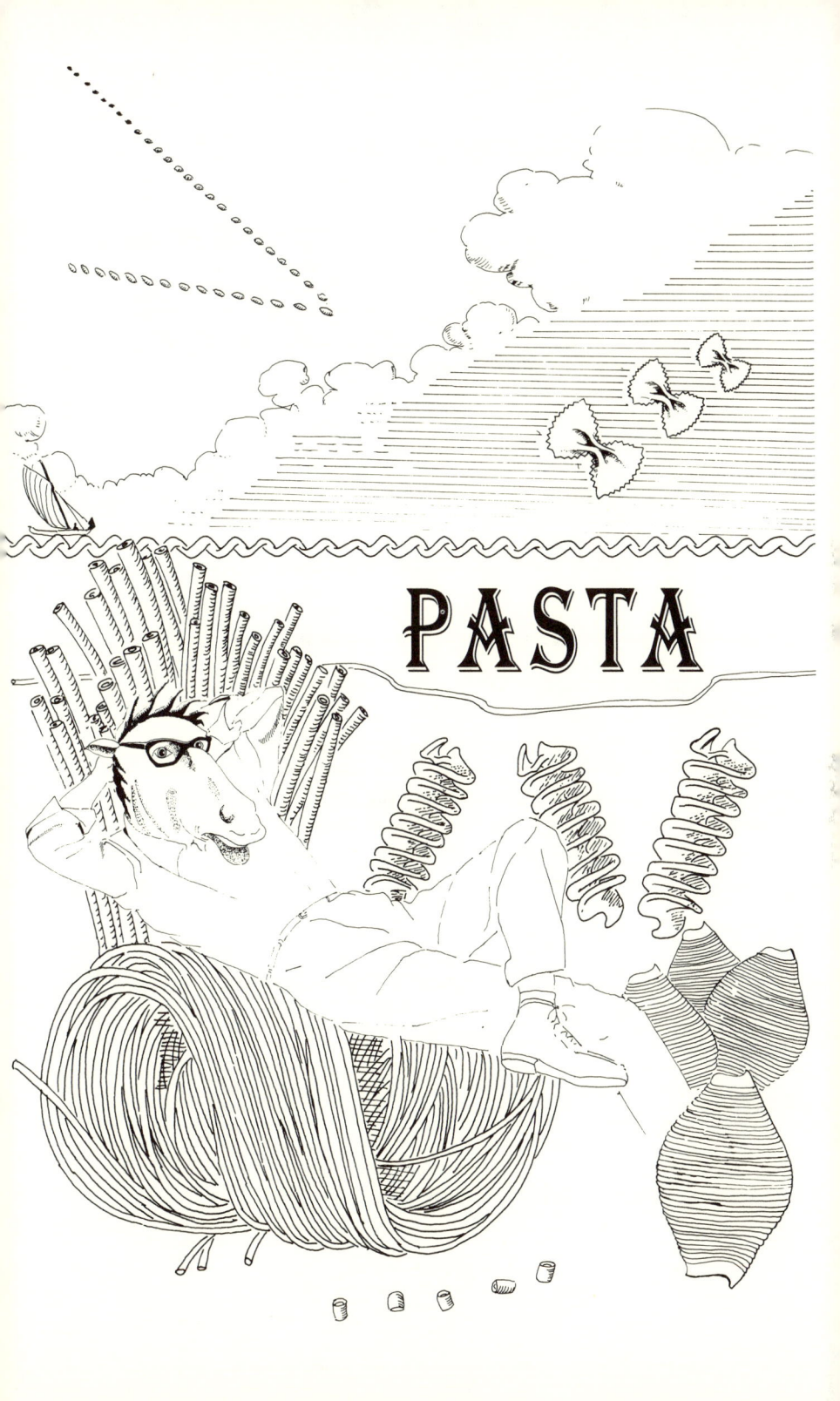

Gorgonzola Lasagna

Serves 8
9 grams per serving

Whoa! Don't turn that page. Imagine an 11" x 14" casserole dish steaming from the oven, and the air scented with the mingled aromas of creamy gorgonzola cheese, mushrooms, and spinach layered with pasta in a hearty tomato sauce.

- 1 lb. lasagna pasta
- ¼ lb. prosciutto (about 8-10 slices)
- ¼ lb. gorgonzola
- 1 10-oz package frozen chopped spinach, thawed
- 1 24-oz carton nonfat ricotta or fat-free cottage cheese
- 1 4.5-oz jar mushrooms, drained
- 4 cups homemade tomato sauce or store bought

Cook pasta in 2 batches, according to package directions. You will need 16 strips. (It's always a good idea to cook a couple of extra strips should one or two break during cooking.) Drain pasta and place on a clean dish towel.

Crumble the gorgonzola and put it in a food processor with the ricotta or cottage cheese; pulse until well-blended. Cover the bottom of the lasagna pan with 1 cup tomato sauce. Place 4 pasta strips over the sauce. Spoon half of the cheese mixture over the strips, smoothing with your fingers. Cover with 4 strips pasta.

Ladle ½ cup tomato sauce over the layer. With scissors, trim the prosciutto of any visible fat and place the prosciutto in a single layer. Put the spinach (squeezed of excess water) over the prosciutto, then the mushrooms over the spinach. Finish this layer with ½ cup tomato sauce.

Put 4 strips over the last layer. Smooth the remaining cheese over the pasta. Cover with the last 4 strips of pasta. Ladle 1 cup of tomato sauce over the lasagna.

Cover with foil, and bake 45 minutes at 350°. Remove the foil and bake 15 additional minutes. Serve with remaining sauce.

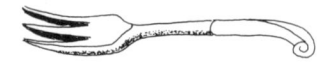

Crock Pot Pasta Sauce

Serves 8
1.2 grams per serving

A very thick and tasty vegetarian tomato-based sauce for pasta. Assemble the night before or in the morning, then let the crock pot do the rest. The carmelized onion gives the sauce its rich and unique flavor.

>2 tsps butter
>1 large white onion, cut in half, then sliced
>2 tsp sugar
>1 28-oz can crushed tomatoes in puree
>3 small zucchini, chopped
>2 carrots, cut into small dice
>1 green pepper, cut in small dice
>2-3 cloves garlic, pressed
>1 Tbs balsamic vinegar
>¼ cup wine or dry Vermouth
>2 Tbs Italian seasoning (or 1 bay leaf, pinch rosemary, 1 Tbs basil, 2 tsp oregano)
>salt, to taste, and ground pepper

Melt the butter in a non-stick sauté pan. Add onion and 1 tsp sugar, stirring until the onion is coated. Sauté for about 10 minutes, stirring frequently over medium-high heat until the onion is a deep golden color.

Put all the remaining ingredients in a crock pot. Add the carmelized onion and cook on low heat for several hours.

Serve over ziti, rotelle (corkscrews), or farfalle (bows).

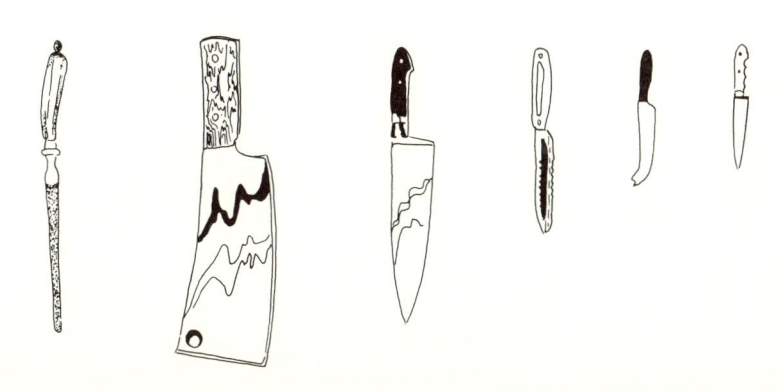

Tuna Pasta Salad

Serves 6
2.3 grams per serving

A new twist on an old standby.

Pasta and vegetables:
1 lb. small macaroni shells
1 Tbs balsamic vinegar
1 12-oz can water-packed tuna
1 cup green peas
2 roasted red peppers, diced, or 1 jar pimentos, drained
½ cup onion, diced

Dressing:
1 cup lowfat cottage cheese
2 Tbs lemon juice
2 tsps dried dill weed
Tabasco, to taste
salt and ground pepper, to taste
2 Tbs fresh parsley, chopped

Cook shells according to package directions. Drain in a colander and rinse under cold water until pasta is cool.

Place pasta in a mixing bowl and toss with vinegar. Add tuna, peas, roasted peppers or pimentos, and onion.

In a food processor or blender, process cottage cheese, lemon juice, dill, and Tabasco until creamy. Season with salt and pepper, to taste. Pour dressing over the tuna pasta mixture and stir. Garnish with parsley. Serve cold.

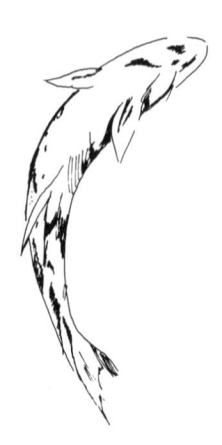

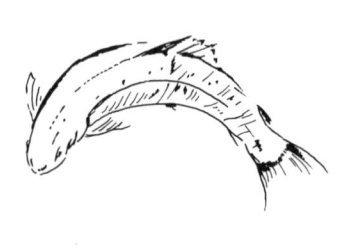

Spinach Fettuccine with Lemon Ricotta Sauce

Serves 4
5.3 grams per serving

Try this if you dream of cream. The sauce can be prepared while the water is boiling for the pasta.

>   1 lb. green fettucine
>   2 cups nonfat ricotta (or 1 15-oz. carton)
>   ¼ cup skim milk
>   ¼ cup white wine
>   1 egg
>   1 Tbs fresh lemon juice
>   1 scant tsp lemon zest
>   salt and pepper, to taste
>   ½ cup shredded hard cheese, like pecorino, asiago, romano or parmesan
>   ¼ cup fresh basil leaves, chopped

Begin cooking pasta according to package directions. Also, bring the water in a double boiler to a rolling boil.

Put the ricotta, skim milk, white wine and egg into the work bowl of a food processor. Process until smooth and creamy. Add the ricotta mixture to the top pot of the double boiler. Whisk in the lemon juice and zest, stirring constantly. Season with pepper and salt. Reduce heat. A couple of minutes before draining the pasta, stir in the grated cheese.

Toss the pasta with the sauce. Garnish with basil leaves and serve immediately.

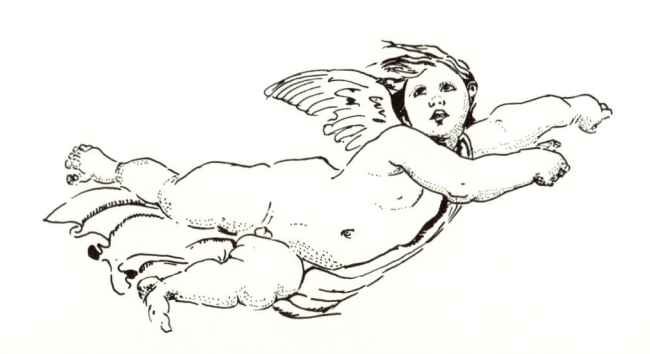

Fettuccine Alfredo with Crab

Serves 4
5.3 grams per serving

This is a recipe to get excited about! Quick, easy, and sumptuous. The sauce is made with Knorr Alfredo sauce mix. Zeb talked to a nutritionist at Knorr and got the low-down: The entire package contains just 11 grams of fat when prepared with skim milk.

- 1 pound fettuccine
- 1 package Knorr Alfredo sauce mix
- 1 cup skim milk
- ¼ cup white wine
- 1 cup crabmeat
- 1 small jar sliced mushrooms
- 2 whole pimentos, diced
- 3 scallions, sliced
- ½ cup green peas

Cook fettuccine according to package directions.

Meanwhile, bring the water in a double boiler to a rolling boil. Reduce heat under double boiler and add to the top pan Alfredo mix and skim milk, stirring with a whisk until the sauce is thickened. When thick, stir in white wine, crabmeat, mushrooms, pimentos, scallions and green peas. Heat through.

Place fettuccine on a serving plate. Cover with the sauce and lightly toss at the table. Serve immediately.

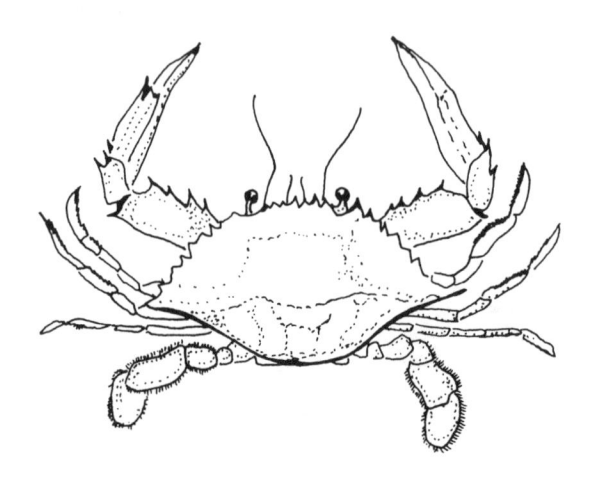

Tuna Creole with Angel Hair Pasta

Serves 4
3.5 grams per serving

The vodka in this easy-to-prepare dish gives it a nice kick. Wine or dry Vermouth may be substituted.

    1 28-oz can crushed tomatoes
    1 large onion, cut in strips
    1 green pepper, peeled and cut in 1"-squares
    1 red pepper, peeled and cut in 1"-squares
    2-3 ribs celery, cut in ½" pieces
    1 large can (12 oz.) water packed tuna, drained
    2 Tbs capers
    1 tsp thyme
    generous dash Tabasco
    1-2 cloves garlic, minced
    8 sprigs parsley (mince 4, reserve other 4 for garnish)
    salt and pepper, to taste
    ¼ cup vodka
    1 lb. angel hair pasta

Place tomatoes and vegetables in large sauce pan. Simmer on medium heat until vegetables are cooked al dente.

Boil water for pasta. Meanwhile, stir the following ingredients into the veggie mixture: tuna, capers, thyme, Tabasco, garlic, parsley, salt and pepper, and vodka. Cook until heated through.

Cook pasta according to package directions, about 3 minutes.

Drain pasta and arrange on a platter. Ladle the Creole over the pasta, garnish with parsley and serve immediately.

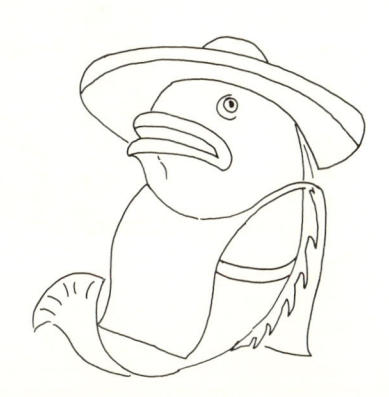

Salmon Pasta Salad

Serves 4
9 grams per serving

Shells and salmon smothered in horseradish dressing is a special favorite of Zeb's. Fat content of salmon varieties varies widely, for example, a pound of Chinook has 47.4 grams while a pound of Chum contains 17 grams. We have used the mean of 32 grams per pound in determining fat content.

    8 oz small pasta shells
    ¾ cup nonfat plain yogurt
    1 Tbs horseradish
    1 lb. cooked salmon (skinned and boned) or 1 17-oz can
    1 Tbs each minced parsley, chives
    2 scallions, chopped
    ½ cup green peas
    1 rib celery, chopped (optional)
    salt and pepper, to taste
    1 tsp paprika

Cook the shells according to package directions. Drain shells in a colander, then rinse under cold water until cool. In a medium bowl, mix together the yogurt and horseradish, combining well. Stir in the remaining ingredients. Place in a serving bowl and refrigerate until well chilled.

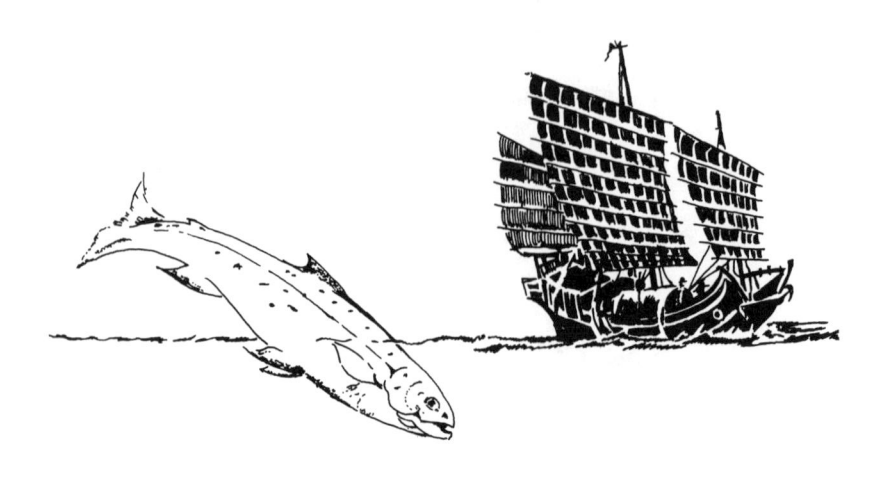

Turkey Tetrazzini

Serves 6
8.6 grams per serving

1 cup celery, chopped
1 tsp butter
12 oz rotini or similar pasta
1 clove garlic
2 tsp dried basil
1½-2 cups cooked turkey
1 jar pimentos or 2 roasted peppers, diced
½-¾ cup green peas
1 jar mushrooms
1 cup grated hard Italian cheese like parmesan, asiago or romano
¼ cup seasoned bread crumbs

Sauce:
1 can lowfat turkey gravy
juice from mushrooms
½ cup dry white wine

Preheat oven to 350°. "Sweat" the celery by cooking it with butter until limp in a small sauté pan. Cook pasta *al dente*. In a 2-cup measure, mix sauce ingredients. Drain pasta and put it in a large oven-proof casserole dish. Press garlic over pasta and stir in basil. Pour sauce over pasta and stir to blend.

Add turkey, celery, pimento or red pepper, green peas, mushrooms, and half of the cheese to the pasta, blending well.

Top with bread crumbs and remaining cheese. Cover and bake for 45 minutes. Remove cover to brown crumbs and cheese, and cook for an additional 5 minutes.

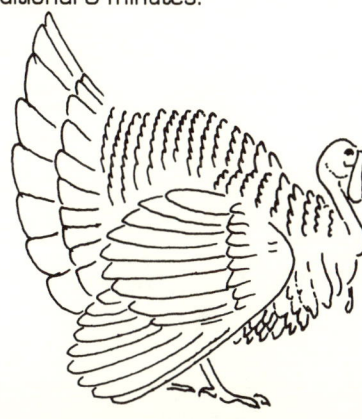

Rigatoni with Mushroom Sauce

Serves 4
6.7 grams per serving

1 Tbs olive oil
1 onion, chopped
1 carrot, chopped
2 celery ribs, chopped
½ cup beef broth
½ cup red wine
1 6-oz can tomato paste
1 lb. mushrooms, sliced
1 clove garlic, minced
1 tsp dried sage
1 19-oz can garbanzo beans
salt and pepper, to taste
1 lb. rigatoni
¼ cup Italian parsley, chopped
2 oz parmesan cheese, grated

Heat oil in a large skillet. Add onions, carrots and celery. Cover and cook over medium-low heat until tender, about 10 minutes. Add to pan beef broth, red wine, tomato paste, mushrooms, garlic and sage. Cook uncovered over medium heat, stirring occasionally, until thickened, about 10-20 minutes. (If too thick, add water.) Stir in garbanzo beans and cook until heated through, about 3 minutes.

Cook rigatoni according to package directions. Drain and toss with sauce; sprinkle with parsley and cheese.

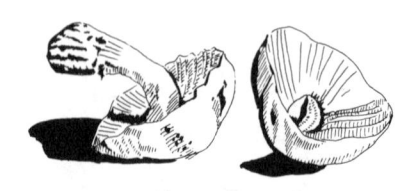

Pasta Primavera

Serves 4
11.3 grams per serving

Don't be daunted by the long list of vegetable ingredients, any combination of the vegetables will create a satisfying meal. Use restraint when steaming the veggies, part of the charm of this dish is its bright spring colors and crunchy texture.

Primavera ingredients:
1 lb. linguine or spaghetti
1 cup each: Fresh diced, corn kernels, broccoli florets, fresh asparagus pieces, snow peas or sugar snap peas, zucchini
1 tsp olive oil
1 medium tomato
½ cup mushrooms, sliced
red pepper flakes, to taste
2-3 large cloves garlic, minced or pressed
3 Tbs. fresh basil, or 1 Tbs dried

Sauce ingredients:
1 Tbs butter
1 Tbs dry Vermouth, optional
salt, to taste
2 Tbs flour
1 cup skim milk
½ cup chicken broth
5 Tbs grated hard cheese

Boil water for pasta. Steam (or blanch) the vegetables. Keep them warm and covered in a slow oven until ready to use. In a non-stick skillet, add the olive oil, tomatoes, mushrooms, red pepper flakes and garlic. Cook for about 5 minutes on medium-low heat.

Cook the pasta according to package directions. Meanwhile, prepare the sauce. Melt the butter in a small saucepan, add 1 Tbs Vermouth and stir well. Add the flour and whisk until the roux is thickened. Add milk, salt and broth, stirring constantly until sauce thickens. Stir in cheese, remove from heat when it is melted.

Place the pasta on a large platter and add all the vegetables. Cover the pasta and vegetables with the sauce. Sprinkle basil on top. Serve immediately, tossing the Primavera at table.

Gnocchi with Pork and Carrots

Serves 4
6.5 grams per serving

Don't knock gnocchi! When you're really hungry, nothing is more satisfying than a hot steaming dish of gnocchi...well, almost nothing. And at 1.5 grams total fat per 15-oz package, you can sate yourself. In this dish, gnocchi are sweetly teamed with pork tenderloin and carrots.

- 1 lb. pork tenderloin, cubed
- 2 large carrots, peeled and cut in 1" chunks
- 3 cups prepared Italian-style tomato sauce
- 1 tsp oil
- ¼ cup red wine (optional)
- salt and pepper, to taste
- ½ tsp dry basil
- 1 15-oz package frozen gnocchi or potato dumplings

Do not defrost gnocchi. In a skillet, brown the pork in the oil. Steam the carrots in a vegetable steamer.

In a large sauce pan, add the tomato sauce, browned pork and steamed carrots. Add the wine, if desired, salt, pepper and basil. Cook on medium heat, until the pork is cooked (about 20 minutes). Meanwhile, cook the gnocchi according to package directions. Drain, and add to sauce. Stir gently and serve immediately.

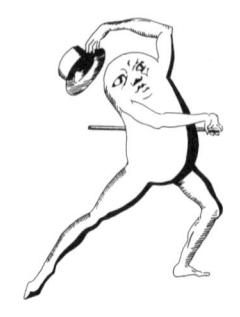

Shells Florentine

Serves 4
8 grams per serving

Recipe can be doubled.

½ package, or 24 large macaroni shells
4 cups tomato sauce
2 egg whites
2 cups nonfat ricotta (approx. 18 oz)
4 oz (1 cup) shredded asiago
1 10-oz package frozen chopped spinach, thawed
½ tsp salt and pepper
¼ tsp ground nutmeg

Cook shells according to package directions, drain and reserve. Preheat oven to 375°. Spoon 2 cups tomato sauce on bottom of a lasagna or similar pan.

In a large mixing bowl, blend together the egg whites, ricotta and asiago. Squeeze excess moisture from the spinach. Add the spinach to the cheese ingredients and combine well. Season with salt, pepper and nutmeg. Using a tablespoon, fill each shell with the cheese-spinach mixture. Arrange stuffed shells in the pan. Cover with foil, and bake for 30 minutes. Remove foil, add the remaining tomato sauce and continue baking for an additional 10 minutes.

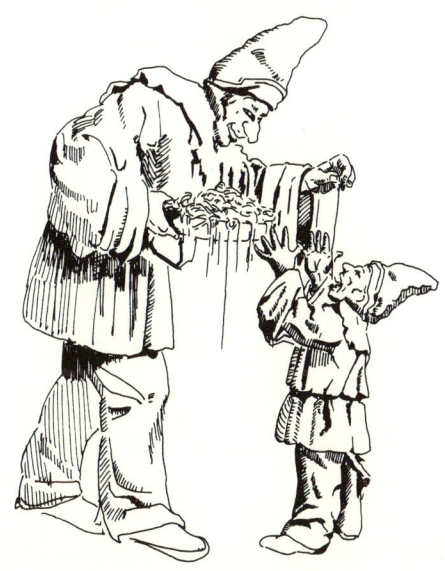

Tubetti in Ricotta Pepper Sauce

Serves 2
2 grams per serving

Admittedly, this recipe isn't for everyone. But if you've wearied of the routine red sauce, need a no-fat cheese fix and are feeling adventurous, then this is the recipe for you. The sauce takes only 2 minutes to fix.

- 4 oz tubetti
- ¼ cup roasted red peppers (fresh or from a jar)
- ¾ cup nonfat ricotta cheese
- 1 tsp balsamic vinegar
- 1 small garlic clove, mashed
- ½ tsp dried basil, or 2 tsp fresh, chopped
- ¼ tsp salt and pepper

Cook pasta according to package directions. Meanwhile, put the roasted red peppers in a food processor and process until liquefied. Add the ricotta, balsamic vinegar, garlic, basil, salt and pepper. Process the mixture until creamy.

Serve sauce over the pasta and garnish with additional basil, if desired.

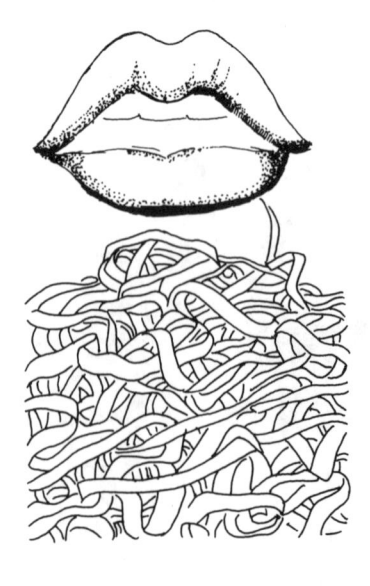

Everything you see I owe to pasta.—*Sophia Loren*

SIDE DISHES

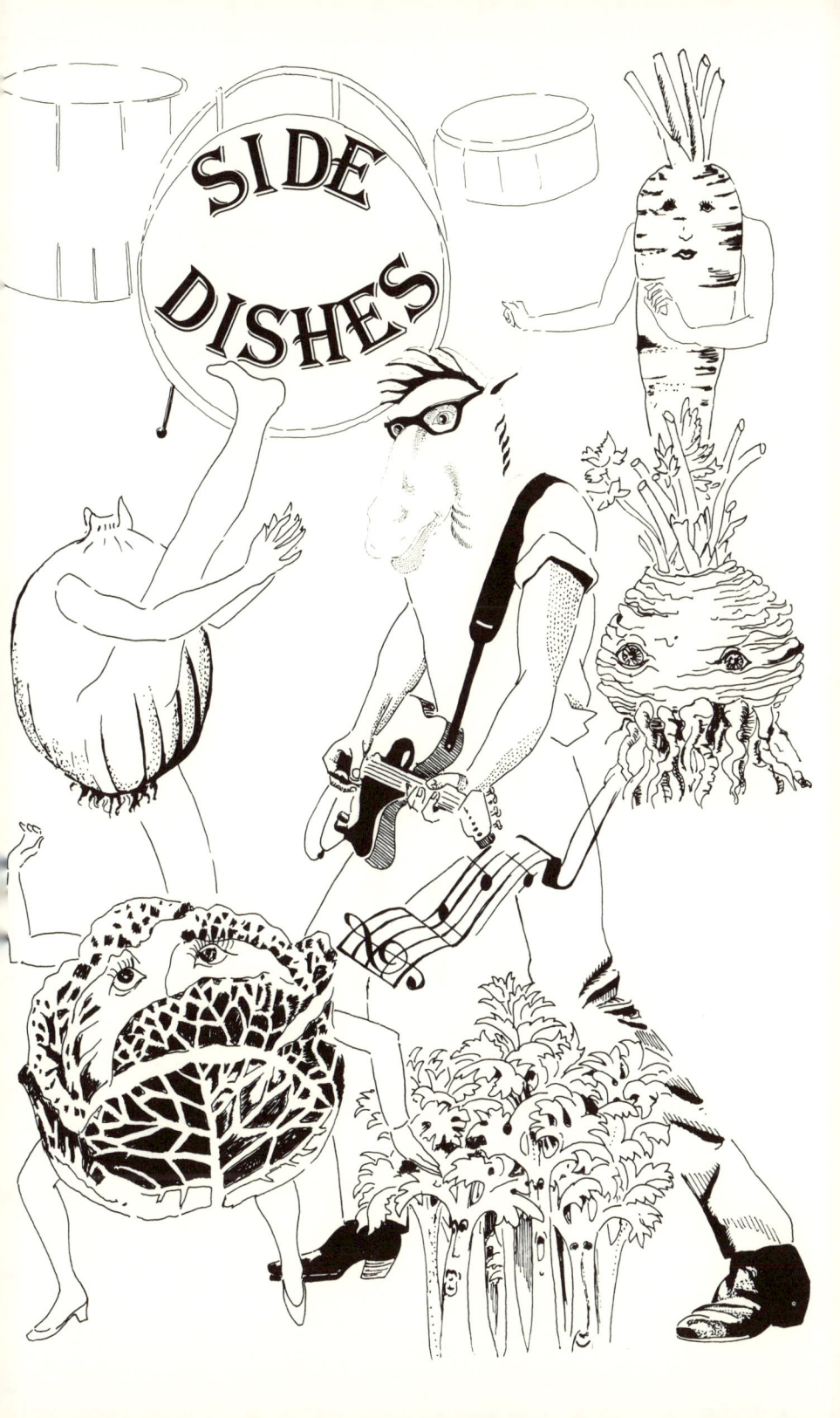

Sesame Seed Green Beans

Serves 4
1.8 grams per serving

- 1 lb. fresh or frozen green beans
- 2 Tbs hulled sesame seeds
- 2 Tbs reduced sodium or lite soy sauce
- 3 Tbs rice vinegar
- 1 Tbs brown sugar

If using fresh beans, wash and trim the ends of the green beans, then cut into bite-sized pieces. Steam until cooked. If using frozen beans, thaw to room temperature.

Brown the sesame seeds in a frying pan. Add soy sauce, rice vinegar and brown sugar to the sesame seeds, and stir to combine. Toss the green beans in the sauce mixture, and cook until heated through.

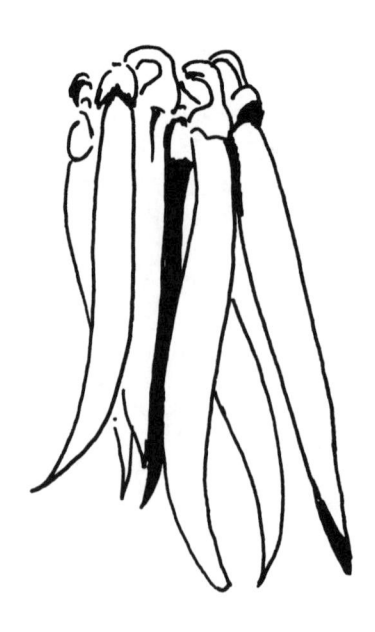

Hungarian Green Beans

Serves 4
3 grams per serving

1 lb. fresh or frozen green beans
6 Tbs sour half & half
2 tsp sweet paprika
½ pound mushrooms, sliced
¼ cup white wine
salt and pepper, to taste

Prepare green beans, as directed in previous recipe. Combine the sour half and half and paprika, set aside.

Put the mushrooms in a large skillet, and sauté them in the wine until cooked. Add the steamed green beans or thawed beans and cook on low heat until the beans and mushrooms are heated through. Before serving, stir in the sour half & half-paprika mixture.

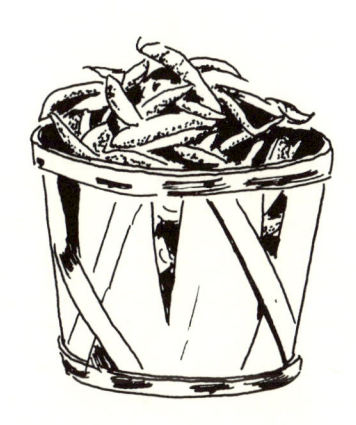

Baked Cauliflower

4 servings
2.7 grams per serving

1 head cauliflower
½ cup skim milk
3 Tbs bread crumbs
¼ tsp nutmeg
¼ cup grated cheese

Preheat oven to 325°. Rinse, core, and remove leaves from a head of cauliflower. Separate into florets. Steam for 6–7 minutes.

In a baking dish, arrange the cauliflower into a mound. Add the skim milk, bread crumbs and nutmeg. Top with cheese and bake for 15 minutes until heated through and lightly browned.

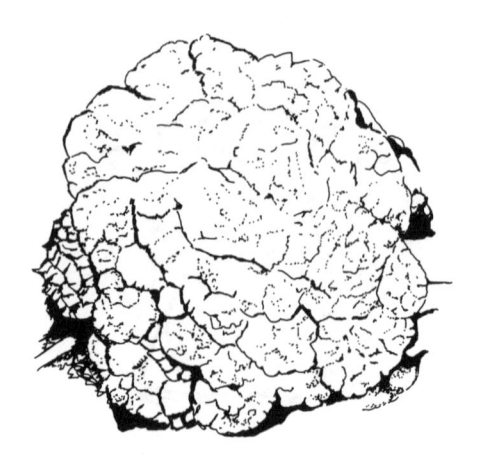

Corn Pudding

Serves 4
3.5 grams per serving

Delicious! And appealing to adults and children alike. The pudding can be assembled and in the oven in five minutes.

    2 cups frozen corn or 15-oz can corn (drained)
    1 12-oz can evaporated skim milk
    2 eggs, beaten
    1 tsp dry mustard
    3 scallions, chopped
    ½ tsp sugar
    ½ tsp salt
    ¼ tsp black pepper
    2 slices, or 1 cup stale white or corn bread torn into bite-size pieces
    ¼ cup diced red pepper or pimento
    skim milk, if needed

Preheat oven to 350°. Mix corn, evaporated skim milk, eggs, mustard, scallions, sugar, salt, pepper, bread and pimento in a medium size mixing bowl. Stir gently until ingredients are blended. Pour pudding mixture into a soufflé bowl. Add milk if pudding does not form a smooth surface on top.

Bake uncovered for 45 minutes to 1 hour, until pudding is set and slightly browned on top.

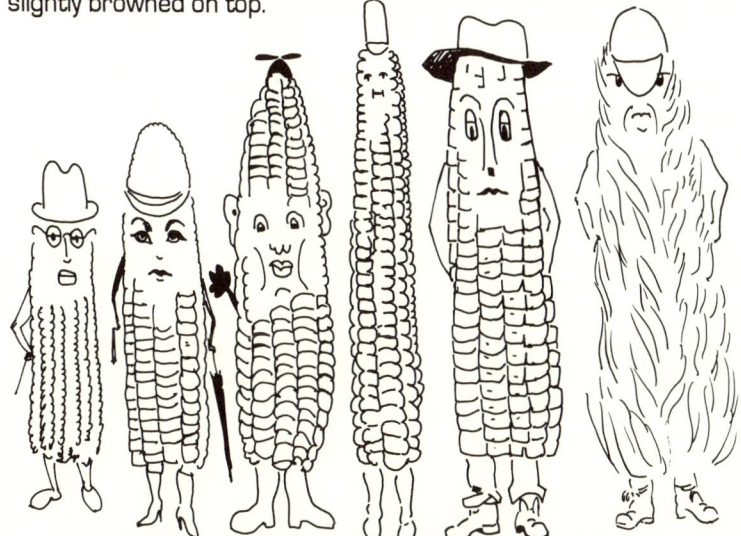

Couscous Primavera with Currants

Serves 6
2.5 grams per serving

A delectable side dish for a party, curried couscous is worth the 3-step program. The dressing doesn't contain any oil, so it is essential that it be added just prior to serving. Otherwise the salad will taste soupy. But for taste, color, and crowd appeal it's a winner!

Step One
2½ cups water
1½ cups instant couscous
½ tsp salt
2 tsp curry powder
fresh ground pepper

Bring water to a boil in a 4-quart pot. Add couscous, salt, curry powder, and pepper. Stir gently. Remove couscous from heat. Cover and let stand for 10 minutes. Fluff with a fork.

Step Two
½ cup carrots, small dice
½ cup broccoli (Cut stalk into match sticks and florets into bite-size pieces)
½ cup red pepper, cut in matchstick pieces
1 scallion, chopped
¼ cup almond slivers
½ cup currants

Put couscous into a serving bowl. Add vegetables, currants and almonds to couscous. Toss with a spatula.

Step Three
Juice of 1 orange
¼ cup dry white wine
1 tsp Dijon-style mustard
1 tsp curry powder

Mix dressing ingredients. Place in a jar and shake. Refrigerate dressing. Prior to serving, pour over couscous and toss.

Simply Scrumptious Creamy Potato Salad

Serves 4-6
0 grams per serving

Friends are always surprised that this potato salad contains zero fat. More than lending curry flavor, the yellow curry powder tricks the palate into thinking the dressing is composed of the standard hard cooked egg-based recipe.

> 4 large boiling potatoes
> ¾ cup nonfat yogurt
> 1 Tbs curry powder
> 1 Tbs Dijon-style mustard
> salt and pepper, to taste
> 2-3 ribs celery, diced
> ¼ cup parsley, minced
> 2-3 Tbs capers
> 2 scallions, chopped
> ½ diced roasted or fresh red pepper (optional)

Bake or boil the potatoes until tender. When cool, peel skins and slice into bite-size dice.

In a large bowl, mix together yogurt, curry powder, and mustard. Add potatoes and remaining ingredients, and gently toss.

Serve very cold.

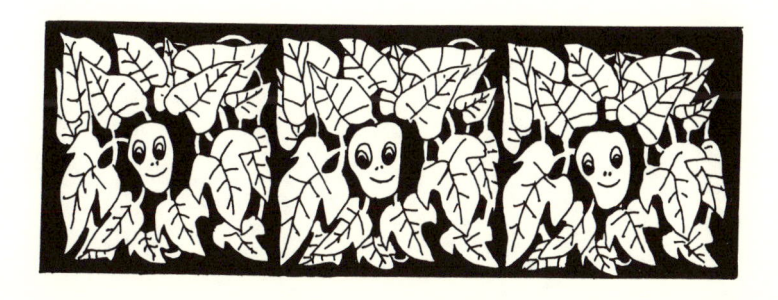

Twice-Baked Potatoes

Serves 2
7.5 grams per serving

A breeze to make if the potatoes are baked the night before, or when the oven is already heated for another purpose.

    2 large baking potatoes
    ½ cup shredded cheese (asiago, or similar cheese)
    ¼ cup skim milk
    ¼ tsp salt and pepper, to taste
    2 Tbs chopped scallion *or* 1 Tbs chives
    1 tsp paprika
    cooking spray

Scrub potatoes, pat dry and bake in a 350° oven for 60 minutes until done. A toothpick inserted in the center should meet no opposition. Set aside to cool.

Cut potatoes in half lengthwise and gently scoop out the potato flesh, taking care not to pierce the jackets. Spray a dish with cooking spray and place the skins in it.

Put the potato flesh in a food processor and pulse 5 times. Add skim milk and cheese and process until mixture is combined (about 10 seconds).

Fill each jacket with one-fourth of the potato mixture. Dust the potatoes with paprika and sprinkle chives or scallions on top.

Bake the potatoes for 30 minutes at 350°, or until hot and slightly browned.

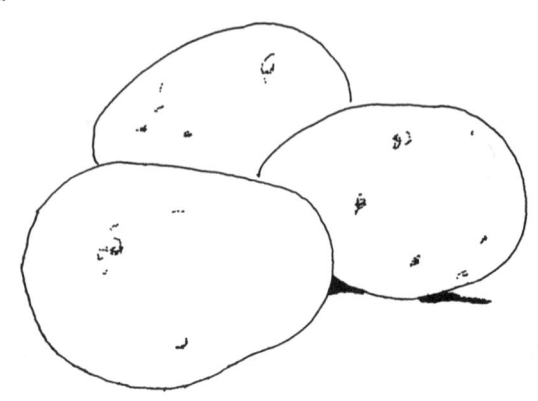

Baked Artichokes

Serves 4
3.7 grams per serving

The twenty minutes this dish takes to prepare is well worth the effort. You'll never want to dunk your artichokes in butter again.

    3 artichokes
    1 lemon, quartered
    2 cloves garlic, peeled and cut in slivers
    2 Tbs red wine vinegar
    1 Tbs olive oil
    2 Tbs dried basil
    ¼ tsp salt
    fresh ground pepper
    ¼ cup water

Heat oven to 400°. To prepare artichokes, cut off stems, pull off the tough bottom row of leaves, and lop ½" off the tops. Quarter artichokes, and with a paring knife remove the fuzzy middle. Rub with lemon. Place artichokes in a baking dish, cut side up. Insert garlic slivers between the leaves. Drizzle vinegar, then oil over artichokes and sprinkle with basil, salt and pepper.

Add water to bottom of pan.

Cover pan with foil, and bake for 35 minutes. Remove from oven and let sit, covered, for 5 minutes. Serve warm or cold.

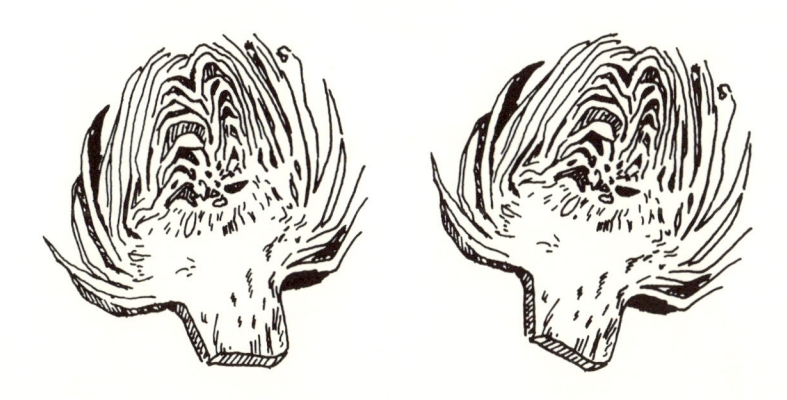

Orzo with Herbs

Serves 4
2.7 grams per serving

Very tasty. For an outstanding variation, substitute the orzo with two cups cooked brown and wild rice.

- 1 cup orzo
- 2 Tbs chopped chives
- 2 Tbs chopped scallions
- 1 Tbs minced fresh parsley
- ¼ cup dry white wine, chicken broth or Vermouth
- ¼ cup shredded parmesan or similar hard cheese
- salt and pepper, to taste

Bring 4 quarts water to a boil. Add orzo and cook on moderately high heat for approximately 8 minutes. Drain pasta and place in an oven-proof or microwaveable casserole dish.

Mix in the remaining ingredients. Keep warm in a slow oven (275°) until serving time. Or heat in the microwave on low setting for 2 minutes.

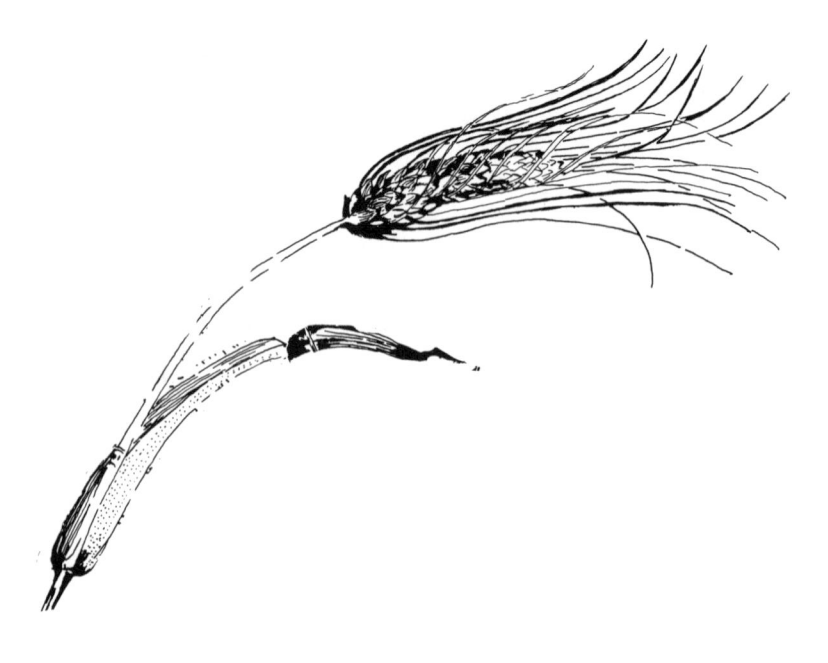

Spanish Rice

Serves 4
3.5 grams per serving

There are many versions of Spanish rice. The recipe below is a purely American concoction, and this rendition is of the empty-out-your-refrigerator variety. Use any combination of vegetables. For best results, use day-old cooked rice.

    1 Tbs olive oil
    1 zucchini, diced
    1 onion, diced
    1 green pepper, diced
    2 cups cooked white or brown rice
    ½ cup corn
    3 Tbs salsa
    2 cloves garlic, crushed
    1 fresh tomato, diced
    ¾ cup tomato juice
    salt and pepper, to taste

Heat nonstick skillet. Add the oil and swirl it around. Add the chopped zucchini, onion, and green pepper, and stir fry until softened.

Reduce heat to medium. Add to the vegetable mixture the rice, corn, salsa, garlic, tomato and tomato juice. Stir well, adding more tomato juice, if necessary. Season with salt and pepper. Serve immediately.

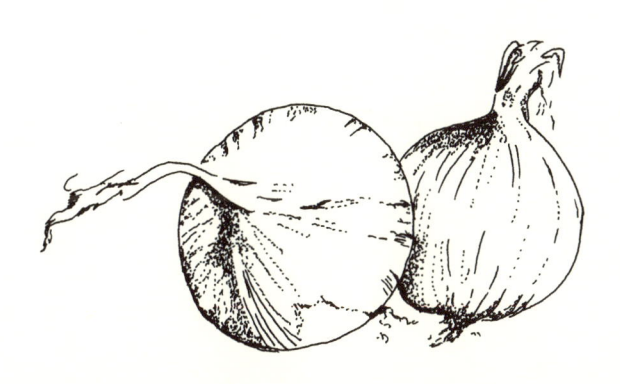

The World's Easiest Spinach Soufflé

Serves 4
2.2 grams per serving

1 16-oz carton nonfat cottage cheese
2 egg whites
1 10-oz package frozen chopped spinach, thawed
¼ cup flour
pinch ground nutmeg
4 Tbs grated hard cheese
salt and pepper, to taste
cooking spray

Preheat oven to 350°. In a medium mixing bowl, beat the cottage cheese until the consistency of cream. Add egg whites, continuing to beat. Squeeze excess moisture from spinach. Fold in the spinach, flour, nutmeg and salt, stirring well until the ingredients are well blended.

Spray a soufflé dish with cooking spray. Place spinach mixture in pan. Top with cheese and bake for 45 minutes until set and crusty on top.

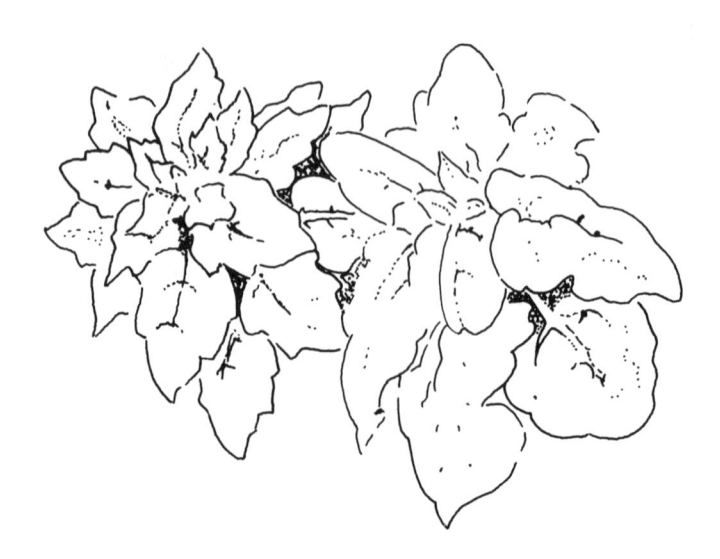

Pintos Rancheros

Serves 6
1.2 grams per serving

1 tsp olive oil
1 cup onions, chopped
1 clove garlic, pressed
1 16-oz can diced tomatoes with liquid
¼ cup green pepper, chopped
1 green chili, minced
1 tsp oregano
salt and pepper, to taste
3 cups cooked pinto beans
½ cup cilantro, chopped

Add the oil, onions and garlic to a large skillet. Sauté the onions and garlic until limp, about 3 minutes. Add tomatoes, green pepper, chili, oregano, salt and pepper. Cook over medium heat for 5 minutes, stirring occasionally. Adjust heat to low and mix in beans. Cook for 10-15 minutes, stirring frequently. Prior to serving, sprinkle with cilantro.

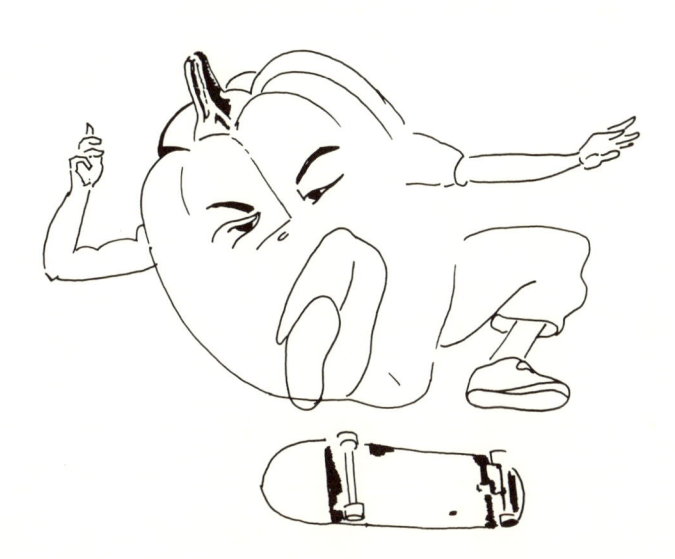

Easy Ratatouille

Serves 4
1.7 grams per serving

Leftover ratatouille makes a great filling for omelets.

- 1 29-oz can tomato puree or crushed tomatoes
- 1 Tbs Italian seasoning, *or* 1 ½ tsp each dried basil, oregano
- 2-3 cloves garlic, minced
- ¼ cup red wine or dry Vermouth
- 1 lb. eggplant, peeled and sliced
- 2 small zucchini cut in ½" disks
- 1 large green pepper, sliced in strips
- 2 medium onions, sliced
- 1 oz or 4 Tbs grated hard cheese

Preheat oven to 325°. Spoon half the tomato sauce into an ovenproof baking dish. Stir in the spices, garlic and red wine or vermouth. Add each vegetable individually, stirring well to incorporate into the tomato sauce. When all the vegetables have been stirred in, top with remaining tomato sauce and toss once more.

Cover with foil; pierce the foil with a fork several times to allow steam to escape. Bake for 90 minutes.

Five minutes prior to serving, sprinkle with cheese.

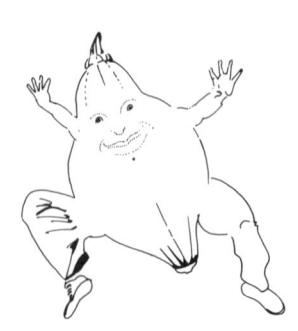

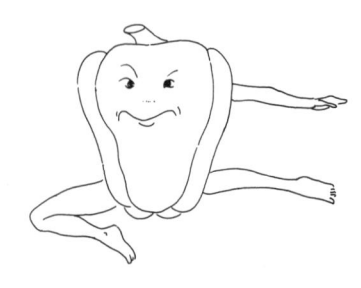

Baked Yellow Rice

Serves 4
2.5 grams per serving

Zeb likes this with roast chicken.

    2 tsps olive oil
    1 cup uncooked rice
    2 cups boiling water
    1 tsp turmeric
    1 tsp salt

Preheat oven to 325°. Coat a 1½ quart casserole with olive oil. Add the rice, boiling water, turmeric and salt. Stir to dissolve turmeric. Cover, and bake for 1½ hours.

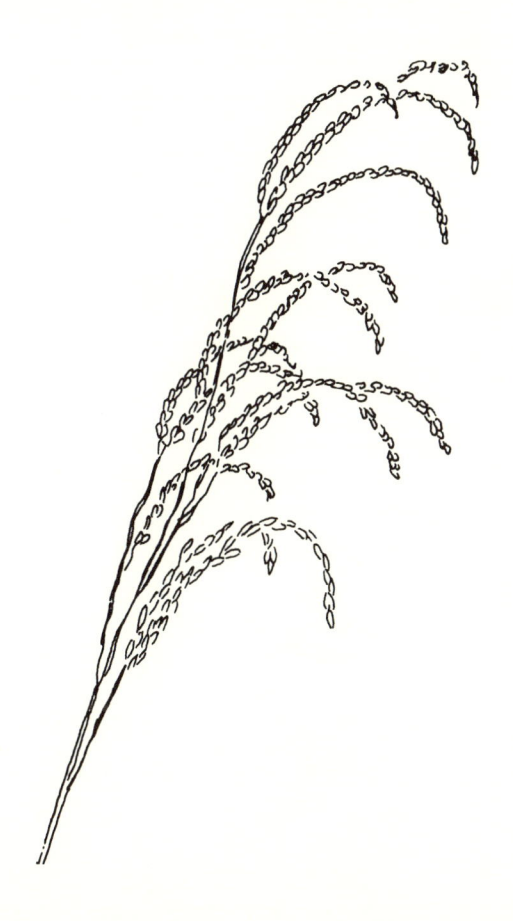

Orange Glazed Carrots

Serves 4-6
0 grams per serving

2 Tbs hot water
1 Tbs cornstarch
½ cup fresh orange juice
¼ tsp ground ginger
4 large carrots, peeled and cut on an angle in 1" chunks

Stir together the hot water and cornstarch until smooth. Into a medium saucepan, add the cornstarch mixture and orange juice. Stir constantly over medium heat until the syrup comes to a boil. Stir in the ginger. Set aside.

Steam the carrots for 7-8 minutes, or until fork tender. Add the steamed carrots to the orange syrup, stirring well.

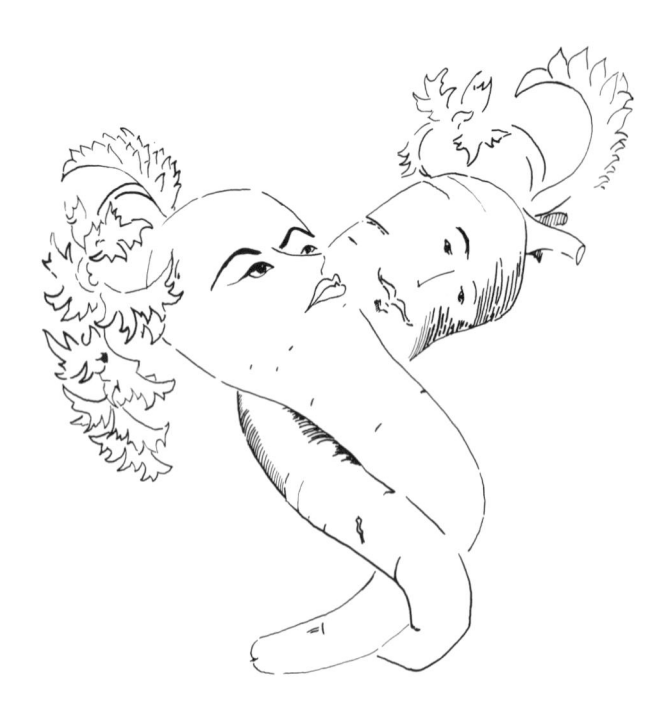

Potato Onion Pie

Serves 6
3 grams per serving

Evocative of the culinary classic *gratin dauphinois*, this potato onion pie is a snap to make—if you have a food processor. If done by hand, the trick is to slice the potatoes and onions uniformly—about an 1/8" thick.

    2 lbs boiling potatoes
    3 medium yellow onions
    salt, to taste, and white pepper
    1 cup skim milk
    ½ cup shredded gruyère or similar cheese

Preheat oven to 350°. Peel the potatoes and process them with the skinniest blade on your food processor. Remove from food processor and immerse in cold water. Peel the skin from the onions, lop in half and send through the food processor using the same blade as you did with the potatoes.

Spray a 9" glass pie plate with cooking spray. Drain a handful of potatoes on a paper towel. Arrange the potatoes on the pie plate. Add a layer of onions, salt and pepper. Continue arranging the potatoes and onions in this fashion until all the potatoes are used, ending with potatoes as the top layer. Pour the milk over the potatoes, tilting the pie plate somewhat so that the milk seeps through the layers.

Cover with cheese and bake for 45 minutes, or until lightly browned and bubbly. Serve in pie-shaped wedges.

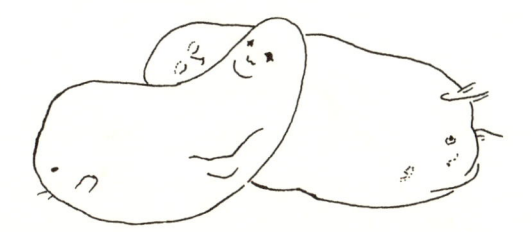

Corn Pancakes

Serves 4
2.2 grams per serving

Fun and easy, the kids can help you make them.

½ cup flour
¼ cup cornmeal
1 Tbs baking powder
½ tsp salt
pepper, to taste
1 egg, lightly beaten
1 10½-oz can creamed corn
cooking spray

In a medium bowl, mix flour, corn meal, baking powder, salt, and pepper. Stir in the egg. Add the creamed corn, mixing well.

Spray a non-stick skillet with cooking spray. Using a tablespoon, drop the batter onto the hot skillet 3-4 at a time. Cook until lightly golden, turn with a spatula and cook the other side. Keep warm in a 250° oven before serving.

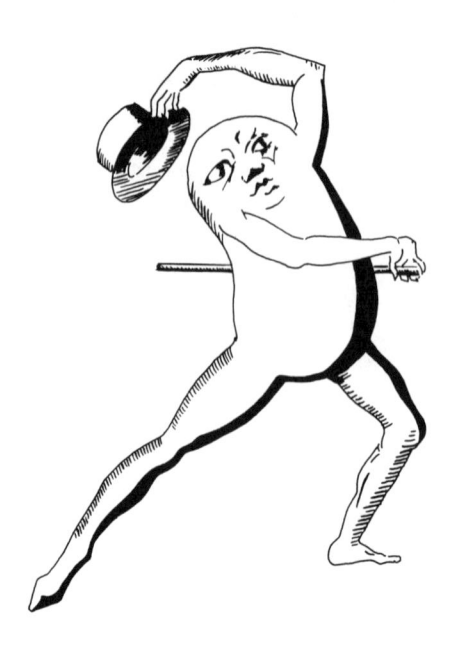

Rosemary Roasted Potatoes in Foil

Serves 6
3 grams per serving

Perfect! No pans to scrub. Simply seal in foil and bake. Use leftovers to fill a 1-yolk omelet.

    1 ½ lbs new potatoes, washed
    3 garlic cloves, pressed or minced
    4 tsps olive oil
    ½ tsp salt
    ¼ tsp each ground pepper and rosemary
    3-4 Tbs chopped fresh parsley

Preheat oven to 375°. Cut the potatoes in half. Put them in a bowl with the rest of the ingredients, except parsley. Stir well to coat evenly and blend flavors.

Place the potatoes in a single layer on 2 sheets foil, or 1 sheet of heavy-duty foil. Place another layer of foil over the potatoes and crimp edges to seal. Bake for 45-50 minutes, until potatoes are tender. Before opening foil, pierce with a fork to allow steam to escape. Sprinkle with parsley.

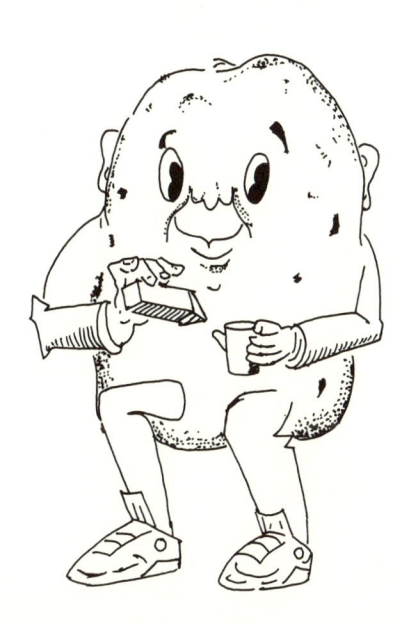

Sweet Potato Pie

Serves 6
1 gram per serving

Try it! A unique combination of flavors and textures. The fiber-rich crust takes just five minutes to prepare and has almost no fat. The ginger-scented sweet potato is whipped into a creamy pie filling that tastes deceptively rich.

Pie crust:
1 ¼ cups cooked brown rice
1 egg, beaten
cooking spray

Sweet potato filling:
1 1-lb. sweet potato, cooked and peeled
¼ tsp ground ginger
1 egg white
½ cup evaporated skim milk
1 Tbs brown sugar
mini marshmallows, for topping (optional)

Preheat oven to 350°. Combine in a bowl the cooked rice and egg, mixing well. Spray a 9" pie pan with cooking spray. With a spatula, spread the rice mixture evenly over the bottom and sides of pan, pressing gently with fingertips.

Bake the crust for about 10 minutes, until set.

Meanwhile, put the cooked and peeled sweet potato in a food processor or blender. Whir until smooth. Add the remaining ingredients, except the marshmallows, and whir until creamy.

Add the filling to the prepared pie shell, dot with mini marshmallows, if desired, and bake at 350° for 35-40 minutes.

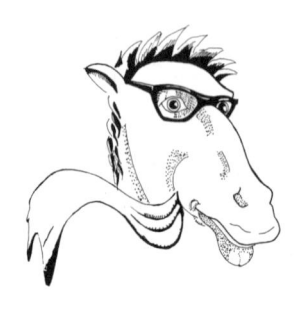

Turmeric Cabbage

Serves 4
2.3 grams per serving

Shredded cabbage rendered vividly golden with turmeric, braised in a little oil and chicken broth is a different take on cabbage. Stuff leftover cabbage with sliced meats into pita pockets.

    1 medium cabbage
    2 tsps veg oil
    ¾ cup chicken broth
    1 tsp turmeric
    salt and pepper, to taste

Remove core from cabbage. Cut cabbage in 8 wedges. Cut each wedge cross-wise in ½" strips or slice in a food processor using the slicing disk.

Swirl the oil in a large non-stick skillet. Add the cabbage, tossing thoroughly over medium heat. When the cabbage begins to wilt, add chicken broth in tablespoon increments and continue stirring until cabbage is cooked. Stir in turmeric, salt and pepper.

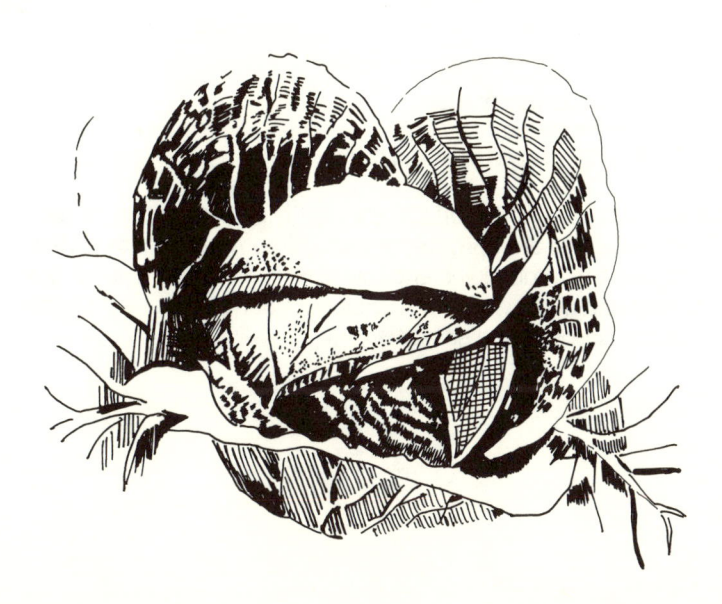

Quick Veggies

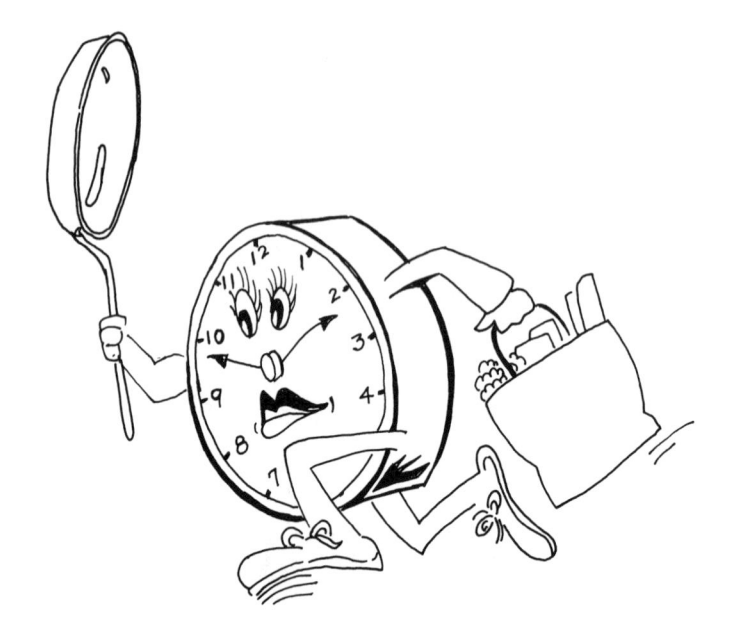

Glazed Brussels Sprouts

Serves 4
0 grams per serving

1 lb. Brussels sprouts
2 Tbs fresh lemon juice
1 Tbs Dijon-style-style mustard

Wash sprouts and lop off the stems. Then cut sprouts in half lengthwise. Steam sprouts for approximately 8 minutes. Meanwhile, put the lemon juice and mustard in a Pyrex measuring cup, stir well and microwave for 1 minute. Pour the sauce over the Brussels sprouts and serve.

Spinach with Chopped Egg

Serves 4
0 grams per serving

1 package frozen chopped spinach, defrosted
2 hard-boiled egg whites, yolks reserved for another use
freshly ground nutmeg
salt and pepper, to taste

Heat spinach in a medium pan. Chop egg whites. Add to spinach. Sprinkle nutmeg, salt and pepper over spinach.

Stewed Tomatoes and Zucchini

Serves 4
0 grams per serving

1 14½-oz can low sodium Italian-style stewed tomatoes
4 small zucchini

Slice zucchini in ¼" rounds. Put in a saucepan with the stewed tomatoes. Heat until zucchini are cooked al dente.

Creamed Corn and Zucchini

Serves 4
0.5 gram per serving

1 8¾-oz can creamed corn
3 small zucchini, sliced in rounds
1 roasted red pepper or ½ small jar pimentos

In a medium sauce pan, heat the creamed corn, zucchini and red pepper or pimento until the zucchini is cooked.

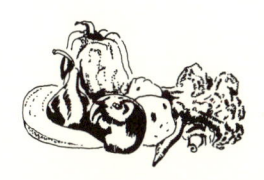

Yellow Squash in Dill

Serves 4
0-Tr. grams per serving

4-6 small yellow squash
1 can low-sodium chicken broth
1 small onion, cut in half rings
2 tsp dill weed

Put all ingredients in a medium sauce pan, and cook until the onion is translucent.

Stir-fried Pea Pods

Serves 4
1.2 grams per serving

1 lb. pea pods
1 tsp sesame seed oil
1 Tbs soy sauce

Snap off the ends and remove strings from pea pods.

Swirl oil in a heated non-stick wok or skillet. Add the pea pods and cook over medium heat stirring constantly until wilted. Add soy sauce and heat for 1 minute more.

Steamed Asparagus

Serves 4
0.6 grams per serving

l lb fresh asparagus, white stalks snapped off
½ cup seasoned bread crumbs
1 whole roasted red pepper, sliced

Steam asparagus until al dente (about 5 minutes). Arrange on a serving dish. Cover with bread crumbs, then top with roasted red pepper. Serve warm or cold.

ENTREES

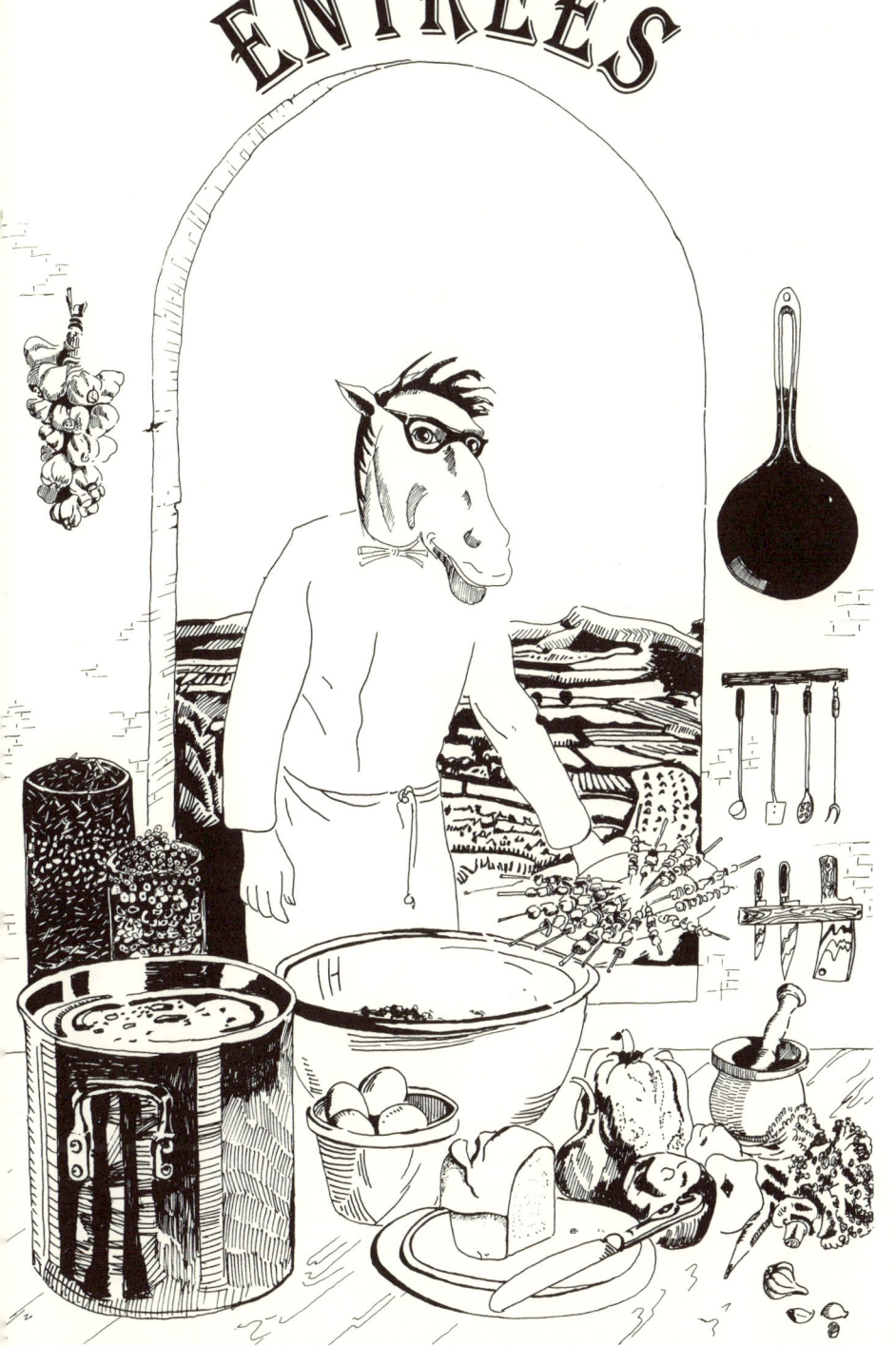

Eat Like a Horse Chicken

Serves 4
6 grams per serving

Hey, you! Try this recipe adapted from Michel Guérard's *Cuisine Minceur*. But, don't eat the hay, it is meant to steam-roast the chicken as well as create a unique presentation.

    2 large handfuls hay (available from stables)
    2 Tbs dried thyme
    1 bay leaf, crushed
    1 3-lb. roasting chicken, skin removed
    salt and pepper, to taste
    ½ cup water

Preheat oven to 425°. Put a layer of hay in the bottom of a lidded casserole. Sprinkle the thyme and crushed bay leaf over the hay. Add the chicken, seasoned with salt and pepper, and cover with another layer of hay. Moisten the hay with the water. Cover and cook for 1 hour.

Bring the chicken to the table in the casserole still surrounded by the hay. Carve the chicken at the table.

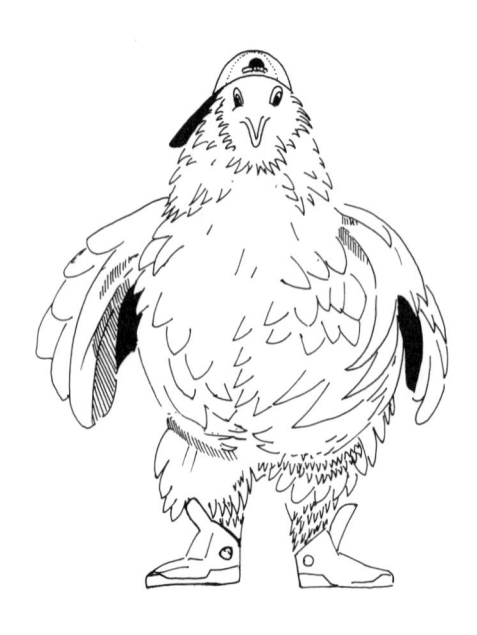

Chicken Yakitori

Serves 4
6.5 grams per serving

Simple to prepare, Japanese chicken kebobs for the grill or broiler. Steamed rice and cucumber raita complete an elegant meal.

    1 Tbs Oriental sesame oil
    2 Tbs rice vinegar or sake
    3 Tbs low sodium soy sauce
    1 clove garlic, crushed
    ¼ tsp ginger powder
    1 bay leaf
    1 tsp sugar
    dash Tabasco
    1½ lbs. skinless, boneless chicken breast
    1 large sweet onion (vidalia or walla walla)
    wood skewers

Mix first 8 ingredients together and place in a medium-sized bowl. Cut the chicken into 1" chunks.

Put the chicken chunks in the marinade, cover with plastic wrap and refrigerate for several hours, or overnight.

Soak the skewers in water for at least 15 minutes. Cut the onion lengthwise into ½" wide strips. Thread the chicken and the onion alternately onto the skewers.

Grill the Yakitori over a low-medium heat, turning every couple of minutes until the kebobs are golden brown and the onion is cooked. Or broil in the oven 4 inches from the source of heat, turning every couple of minutes.

If desired, cook the marinade and use it as a dipping sauce. Bring the marinade to a boil, then simmer gently for 5 minutes. Remove the bay leaf prior to serving.

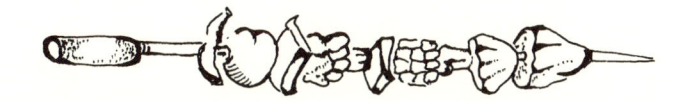

Oven Baked "Fried" Chicken

Serves 4
8 grams per serving

Patrons of fast-food venues will savor the taste of this "fried" chicken. Remember just one piece of fried breast meat the way *they* do it contains 23.7 grams of fat. Using *our* cooking method, 8 pieces of chicken—white and dark meat—weigh in at 32 grams, but we know you wouldn't eat all that chicken by yourself! (The spice mixture yields approximately ¾ cup, or 6 oz, of mix. Store the mix in an air-tight container.)

Spice Mixture:

1 Tbs rosemary	3 Tbs brown sugar
1 Tbs oregano	3 Tbs dried parsley
1 Tbs powdered sage	1 tsp ground pepper
1 tsp powdered ginger	1 Tbs paprika
1½ tsp thyme	2 Tbs garlic salt
	2 Tbs powdered onion

Place all ingredients in a blender or food processor and blend for 1 minute to pulverize.

Chicken ingredients:

1 3-lb. chicken cut in 8 pieces, skin removed	¾ cup flour
1 cup buttermilk	2 Tbs spice mixture

An hour before baking the chicken, place the chicken pieces with the buttermilk in a bowl.

Preheat oven to 375°. Mix together the flour and 2 Tbs of the spice mixture, blending well. Put spice-flour mixture on a plate. Dredge the chicken pieces in it, coating both sides. Spray a cookie sheet with cooking spray and place the chicken pieces on it. Cook for 20 minutes, then turn pieces over and cook for an additional 20 minutes.

Tandoori Chicken

Serves 4
6 grams per serving

This tender and subtly spiced dish can be prepared in 5 minutes if your butcher cuts up and skins the chicken and you use a commercially prepared Tandoori mixture. Sharwoods, available at specialty stores, is a good one. The homemade Tandoori mixture recipe follows.

>   3-lb. fryer cut in eight pieces, skin removed
>   2 Tbs nonfat yogurt
>   Tandoori mixture
>   2 Tbs cider vinegar
>   2 Tbs fresh lemon juice

In a bowl large enough to contain the chicken, mix the yogurt, tandoori spice mixture, vinegar and lemon juice, stirring well to form a paste. Smother the chicken in the paste, turning often to fully coat the chicken pieces. Cover the chicken and marinate at least 8 hours or overnight in the refrigerator.

Before cooking, shake off excess marinade. Broil or barbecue 10 to 15 minutes on each side.

Tandoori Spice Mixture:

>   1 tsp paprika
>   ¾ tsp each salt, turmeric, ground cumin
>   ¼ tsp cinnamon or powdered cloves
>   ½ tsp ground ginger
>   ¼ tsp each black pepper and cayenne
>   2 cloves minced garlic
>   ½ tsp dry mustard

Place the spices in a small bowl, mortar and pestle, or mini food processor and grind the spices well.

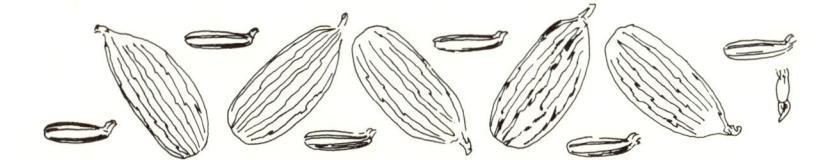

Chicken Piccata

Serves 4
5 grams per serving

This recipe yields a cup of tangy and virtually nonfat sauce. Pour the sauce over new potatoes or angel hair pasta for a great one-dish meal.

1 tsp butter
1 lb. boneless, skinless chicken breasts, halved
1 lemon, sliced in eight circles for garnish
1 14-oz can chicken broth
½ cup dry Vermouth
1 Tbs fresh lemon juice
1 Tbs flour
3 Tbs capers
salt and pepper, to taste

In a nonstick skillet melt the butter. Sear the chicken breasts until nicely browned, but do not overcook. Remove the chicken from the skillet and place in an ovenproof serving dish. Place two lemon circles over each breast. Cover dish with foil and keep warm in a 275° oven.

In the skillet, bring the chicken broth to a boil with the pan juices, allowing the broth to reduce somewhat. Turn the heat down and add the Vermouth and lemon juice. Continue cooking the sauce for an additional 5 minutes. Whisk in the flour until the sauce is thickened. Add capers, salt and pepper to the sauce.

Remove chicken breasts from the oven and pour any pan juices into the sauce, stirring to incorporate. Pour some of the sauce over the chicken and use the rest for pasta or potatoes.

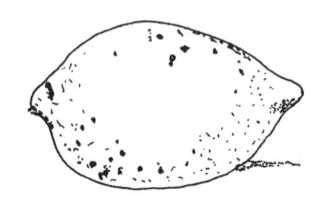

Arroz Con Pollo

Serves 1 or a crowd
13.4 grams per serving (with skin)

This chicken and rice dish is as colorful as a paella, and far less costly—an excellent party entree. Measures are given for one person, for easy multiplication. For more fat savings in your account, don't eat the skin.

    oil for frying (preferably olive oil)
    garlic to taste, up to 3 cloves
    ¼ tsp saffron
    1 chicken breast half
    ½ cup chicken broth
    ¼ cup white wine, *or* 3 Tbs dry Vermouth
    1 cup cooked medium grain rice, kept warm
    ½ red pepper, sliced into strips
    ½ green pepper, sliced into strips
    ½ onion, sliced
    ½ zucchini, sliced in rounds
    1 Tbs Spanish capers
    4-5 green olives
    salt and pepper

In a sauté pan, heat 1 tsp oil. Cut garlic into slivers and gently sauté until limp; remove and set aside. Pinch a few threads saffron into the pan. Sauté the chicken breasts, skin side down until skin turns a golden brown. Remove chicken from the pan and place in a deep pot. Add chicken broth and white wine or Vermouth and gently simmer on low heat, adding garlic and remaining saffron to the pot..

Sauté the red and green peppers, onions and zucchini until lightly browned. Reserve. 10 minutes before serving, place the vegetables on top of the chicken in the pot and add the olives and capers. Reduce heat to low and simmer gently until heated through.

Mound the cooked rice in the middle of a serving platter. Place the chicken and vegetables around the rice. Serve immediately.

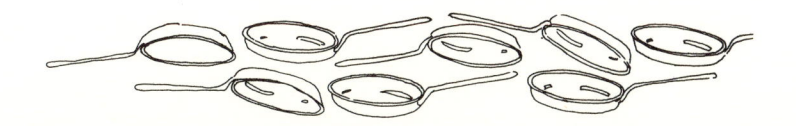

Chicken Cutlets with Rosemary

Serves 4
6.7 grams per serving

2 whole boneless, skinless chicken breasts, split
1 Tbs olive oil
2 Tbs Worcestershire sauce
1 Tbs fresh lemon juice
1 Tbs red wine vinegar
1 tsp rosemary
Tabasco sauce
salt and pepper, to taste

Flatten each chicken breast half into a cutlet. Remove the tendon. Put each breast between 2 sheets waxed paper and flatten to a thickness ¼ inch or less.

Mix oil, Worcestershire, lemon juice, vinegar, rosemary and Tabasco in a nonstick skillet. Heat marinade over high heat. When hot, season chicken with salt and pepper and add to skillet. Cook, turning several times, until lightly browned on both sides and no longer pink inside (about 3 minutes). Serve immediately with pan juices.

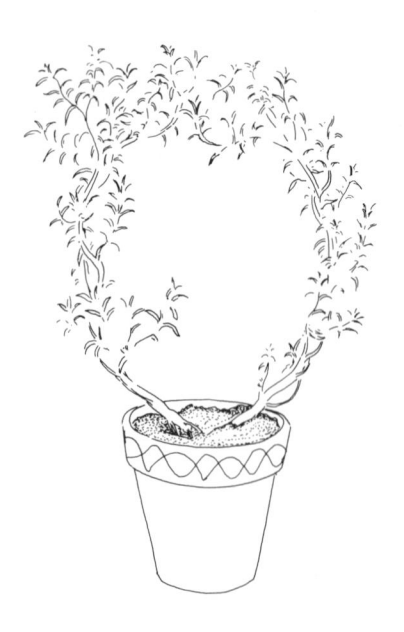

Chicken and Pork Adobo

Serves 4-6
7 grams per serving

A variation on a popular Filipino dish. This version uses boneless, skinless chicken breasts and pork tenderloin without sacrificing its characteristic flavor.

- 1 lb. chicken breasts, cut in nuggets
- 1 lb. pork tenderloin, cut in nuggets
- ½ cup white or cider vinegar
- 1 Tbs soy sauce
- 4-6 cloves garlic, crushed
- 1 bay leaf
- 2 tsp vegetable oil
- white rice

Marinate chicken and pork in vinegar, soy sauce, crushed garlic and bay leaf about 1 hour. Turn at least once.

Sauté chicken and pork in a large skillet with oil until golden brown. Turn frequently to avoid searing meat. Reserve marinade. Remove meat from pan and set aside. Add the marinating liquid to the skillet and heat until boiled. Reduce heat, and add the browned meat. Simmer on medium-low heat for approximately 30 minutes, or until tender.

Place in a serving dish and serve with rice.

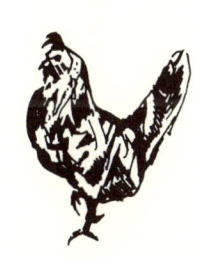

Chicken Fajitas

Serves 4
6.3 grams per serving

The standard marinade for Fajitas calls for up to half a cup of oil. (110 grams, Yikes!). In this variation, cooked chicken is enveloped in a sauce comprised of salsa and sour half & half. Different, quick, and tasty—kids love it. Grill the chicken whenever possible.

1½ lbs. skinless, boneless chicken breasts
Chicken seasoning: 1 tsp each ground cumin, garlic powder, chili powder, dried or fresh cilantro
5 Tbs prepared salsa
3 Tbs sour half and half
4 trimmed scallions, cut lengthwise
¼ cup water
cooking spray
8 flour tortillas

Shred chicken into strips. Put seasoning mixture in a plastic bag, add chicken and shake to coat. In a small bowl, mix together salsa and sour half & half, refrigerate.

Spray a non-stick baking dish with cooking spray. Add chicken and scallions and ¼ cup water. Cover, and cook chicken for 30 minutes at 325°. When done, drain liquids and set aside. Turn off oven and warm the tortillas for 2 minutes.

Place a tortilla on a plate. In the center of the tortilla, spoon 1 Tbs salsa mixture, 3-4 chicken strips and 1 scallion half. Roll into a tube for Fajitas.

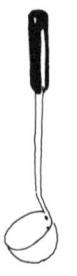

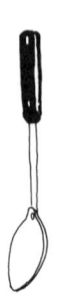

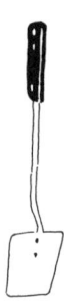

Cheese and Chicken Enchiladas

Serves 4
4 grams per serving

The cheese? No-fat ricotta. These enchiladas are surprisingly easy to make.

Enchilada sauce:
1 8-oz can tomato sauce
3-4 Tbs prepared salsa
¼ tsp ground cumin
½ tsp chili powder

Enchiladas:
1 15-oz tub nonfat ricotta
1 lb. cooked chicken breasts, cut in 1" strips
4 scallions, chopped
8 5" flour tortillas

Preheat oven to 350°. In a small bowl mix together the ingredients for enchilada sauce, stirring well. Spread half the sauce in a 7 ½" x 12" baking pan.

In a medium bowl, combine the ricotta, chicken and scallions. Spoon one eighth of the mixture in the center of the tortilla and roll into a tube. Place enchilada seam side down in the baking pan. Repeat until all the mixture and tortillas are used.

Spoon the remaining sauce over the enchiladas and cover with foil. Bake for 30 minutes. Remove foil and continue to bake for 10 minutes.

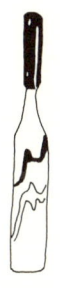

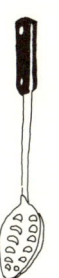

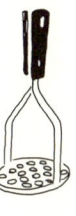

Honey Mustard Chicken

Serves 6-8
4.5 grams per serving

Chicken smothered in a honey-mustard sauce lends itself particularly well to a quick dinner party entree.

- 4 plump chicken breasts (1½ lbs), split in half and skinned
- ½ cup Dijon-style mustard
- ½ cup honey
- 1 tsp dried tarragon
- 2 Tbs soy sauce

Place the chicken snugly in a baking dish. In a small bowl, mix the mustard, honey, tarragon and soy sauce until well combined. Pour mixture over chicken. Cover, and refrigerate for 6 hours or overnight.

Heat oven to 350°. Remove chicken from refrigerator and turn several times. Cover with foil and bake for 45 minutes. Remove the foil and baste well. Uncover, and bake for 5 minutes more. Spoon sauce over chicken.

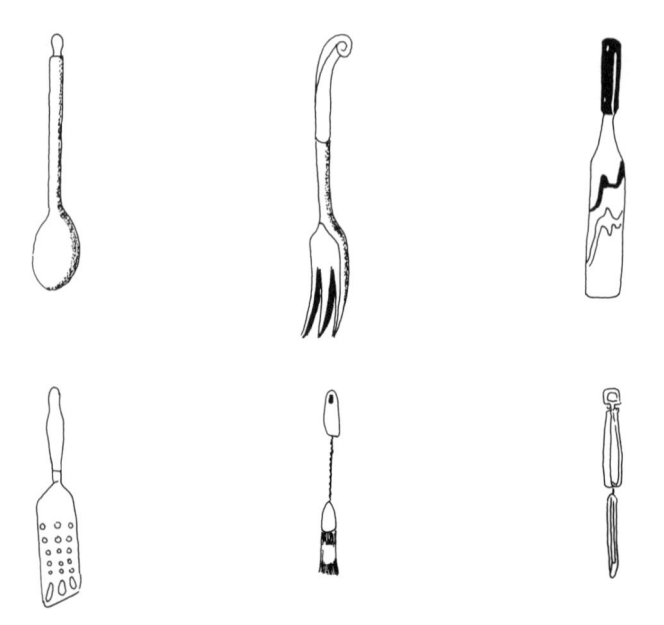

Glazed Game Hens

Serves 4
8.3 grams per serving without skin
14 grams per serving with skin

A sublime recipe for a special occasion.

    2 Cornish game hens
    ¼ cup Amaretto di Saronno, or reasonable substitute

Preheat oven to 350°. With poultry scissors or sharp knife, remove the backbone from the hen. Clean out the cavity, rinsing the bird under cold water. Slit the breast, running the blade down the middle. If done correctly, each piece will have a breast half, leg and wing. Fold the bird in half. If necessary make a cut halfway through the rib to make the fold snug. Lay the bird, wing side down, breast side up in a square Pyrex baking dish. Repeat the procedure with the other hen. Bake for 20 minutes, then drain the fat from the hens.

Ladle the Amaretto on the hens, basting frequently until all the mixture is used. Bake 25 minutes more or until the hens are a crispy golden brown.

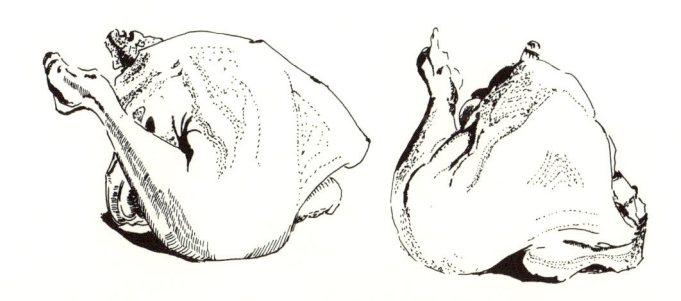

Sweet and Sour Cabbage

Serves 4
5 grams per serving

A one-dish meal similar to stuffed cabbage rolls, but sooo much easier. No big pot of boiling water for blanching cabbage leaves ...just that fabulous flavor that brings back fond memories.

- 1 large onion, chopped
- 1 lb. lean ground turkey (97% fat-free)
- 1 tsp oil
- 1 medium cabbage (about 1 ½ lbs.)
- 1 16-oz can crushed tomatoes
- ½ tsp salt
- ground pepper to taste
- ½ cup raisins
- ¼ cup fresh lemon juice
- ¼ cup honey
- up to 1 ½ cups tomato juice
- 2 cups cooked brown rice

Place the chopped onion and turkey in a large non-stick skillet with the oil. Cook until the turkey is lightly browned. Use a fork to break up large clumps of meat.

Meanwhile, core the cabbage, discarding tough outer leaves. Slice the cabbage into 6 wedges and slice each wedge into 1" wide strips.

Add the onions, browned turkey, cabbage and tomatoes with their juice to a Dutch oven with the salt, pepper, raisins, lemon juice and honey. Simmer for 15 minutes, stirring occasionally, adding tomato juice as needed. Add the rice, cover, and cook for an additional 15 minutes. Adjust seasoning.

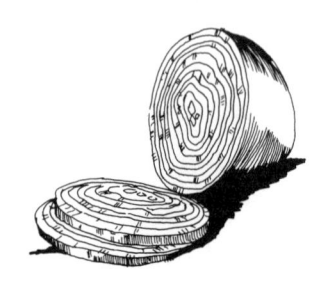

Money Bags

Serves 4
9.8 grams per serving

Steamed meat balls are known in Chinese cuisine as "shu-mei" but we call ours "money bags" because the won ton skins are shaped into little pouches.

> ¾ lb. 93% fat-free ground turkey
> 2 tsp cornstarch
> 1 Tbs dry sherry
> 1 tsp sesame seed oil
> 1 Tbs soy sauce
> ¼ - ½ tsp powdered ginger (use fresh, if available)
> 1 clove garlic, minced
> 2 scallions, chopped
> 1 tsp brown sugar
> 24 won ton wrappers
> cooking spray

In a medium bowl mix together all the ingredients except the won ton wrappers and cooking spray. Blend thoroughly with your hands.

Place a generous tablespoonful of the meat mixture in the center of a won ton wrapper. Fold each point upward so that the four points meet. Squeeze a little of the meat mixture towards the points, then with your fingers crimp the won ton wrapper into a pouch. Flatten the bottom of the pouch gently against the countertop.

Spray the racks of a bamboo steamer with cooking spray. Place the steamer in a pot of boiling water and steam for 20 minutes.

An ordinary vegetable steamer works just as well, but you'll need to cook in 2 batches.

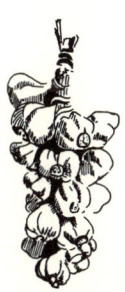

Sloppy Jalopies

Serves 4
8 grams per serving

An American standard popular with kids and adults alike. Rather than use hamburger buns, create "jalopies" out of toasted Italian or French bread.

    1 lb. 97% fat-free ground turkey
    ½ cup chopped onion
    ½ cup catsup
    ½ cup tomato sauce
    1 Tbs Worcestershire sauce
    2 Tbs vinegar
    1-2 tsps Dijon-style mustard
    1 tsp paprika
    1 Tbs brown sugar
    1 large loaf Italian or French bread

In a large non-stick skillet sauté the ground turkey and onion until the turkey is lightly browned and the onion is wilted. Stir in the catsup, tomato sauce, Worcestershire sauce, vinegar, mustard, paprika and brown sugar. Break up large clumps of meat. Cover and simmer on medium heat for 20-30 minutes, stirring occasionally.

Before serving, cut bread in half lengthwise, then in half. Toast the bread under the broiler or in a toaster oven until crisped.

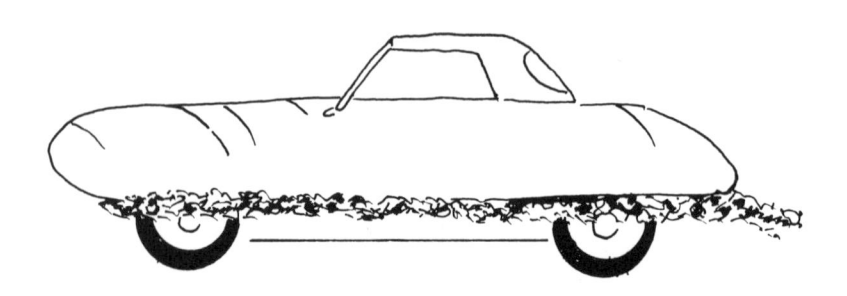

Chili Blanco

Serves 4
4.7 grams per serving

A change from the red stuff, easy to prepare, and tasty—a worthy addition to your culinary bag of tricks.

    2 16-oz cans Great Northern beans, drained of liquid
    ½ lb. cooked and cubed chicken or turkey
    1 can beer
    1 4-oz can diced green chilies
    1 onion and 1 green pepper, diced and sautéed in 1 tsp oil
    2 Tbs fresh cilantro, chopped
    2 cloves garlic, minced
    2 Tbs powdered cumin
    1 Tbs oregano
    red pepper, to taste
    salt, to taste

Put all ingredients in a 4-quart saucepan. Stir and heat through. Serve with hot tortillas.

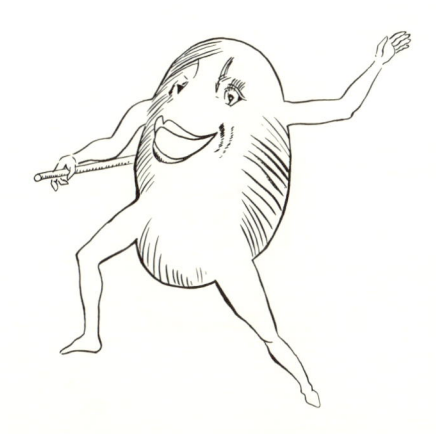

Turkey and Rice Green Pepper Boats

Serves 6-8
3 grams per serving

A hearty one-dish meal that can be prepared as a vegetarian dinner. Simply substitute the ground turkey with a 15-oz can of small red kidney beans (rinsed and drained) and ½ cup corn kernels.

    1 lb. 97% fat free ground turkey
    2 cups cooked brown rice
    1 zucchini, diced
    1 small onion, diced
    minced garlic, to taste
    2 tsp Worcestershire sauce
    salt and pepper, to taste
    2 Tbs Fines herbes or Italian seasoning *or* 1 Tbs any combination of minced fresh parsley, oregano, basil, thyme
    4 green peppers seeded and cut in half lengthwise

Version 1: Preheat oven to 350°. Put all ingredients except peppers in a large mixing bowl. Mix to combine with a big spoon or your presumably clean hands.

Fill peppers with turkey-rice mixture and place in a large baking pan. Add ½" water to the pan. Cover with foil and bake for 90 minutes. Remove foil during last 30 minutes of cooking time.

Version 2: Instead of adding water to the baking pan, add half of a 28-oz can tomato puree to the bottom of the pan. Add stuffed peppers and cover with foil. During last the 30 minutes of cooking time, remove foil and ladle remaining tomato puree over peppers.

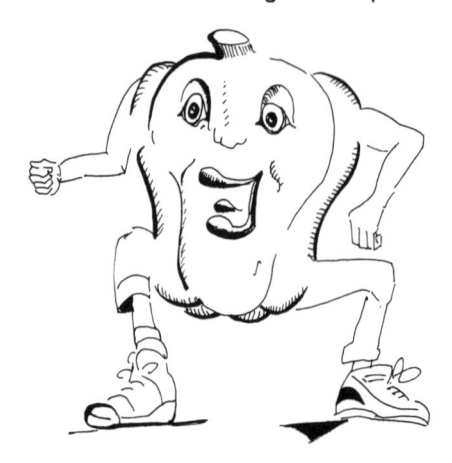

Turkey Picadillo

Serves 10
6.7 grams per serving

This is a festive entree, which never fails to delight a crowd. The picadillo can be made the morning of the event, or even better, the day before. Bake a turkey breast in the oven, reserving the leftover turkey for another recipe in this cookbook. Don't wimp out by using that nasty turkey roll from the deli counter. Fat alert: astute readers will note that one 8-oz jar of olives contains more fat than 2 pounds of white meat turkey breast!

1 5-6 lb. turkey breast
2 28-oz cans whole tomatoes with juice
½ cup white vinegar
salt, to taste and 1 Tbs pepper
¾ tsp cinnamon
1 tsp ground cloves
2 bay leaves
4 cloves garlic, minced
2 onions, chopped
4 green peppers, sliced into strips
2 Tbs peanut or olive oil
1 8-oz jar green olives
¼ to ½ cup Spanish capers
Tabasco
1 cup raisins, plumped in water

Cook the turkey in a roasting pan in the oven according to directions or for 1½-2 hours at 325°. Remove all the meat from one side of the breast, or enough for 10 servings, discarding the skin. Cut the meat into 1" x 1" cubes.

In a crock pot or Dutch oven, add the tomatoes, vinegar, salt and pepper, cinnamon, cloves, bay leaves and garlic. Simmer on a slow heat for 2-3 hours until flavors have mingled.

Sauté the onions and green peppers in oil, set aside.

An hour before serving, add the turkey, onions and green peppers to the sauce, along with the olives, capers, Tabasco and raisins. Heat until the picadillo is piping hot. Adjust the seasoning, adding more cinnamon, cloves, garlic, salt and pepper if necessary. Serve over white rice.

Shrimp Fiesta

Serves 6
2.8 grams per serving

A festive main dish for a party, easily prepared. So low in fat, you can budget a dessert splurge.

> 1 28-oz can crushed tomatoes with puree
> 1 large onion (1 cup)
> 3 ribs celery
> 1 green pepper
> 4 cloves garlic, chopped in a fine dice
> 2 tsp dried cumin
> 2 lbs. raw shrimp (medium or large)
> 1 cup green peas
> 1 15-oz can black beans, rinsed and drained
> ¼ cup white wine (or dry Vermouth)
> 1 tsp Tabasco

Place the tomatoes in a large pot and heat through.

Meanwhile, slice the onion, vertically. Halve the celery up the middle, then slice on the diagonal. Peel the pepper and cut into 1" squares. Add the vegetables, garlic, and cumin to tomatoes. Cook over medium heat until the vegetables are cooked, stirring occasionally. While the vegetable mixture is cooking, peel and devein the shrimp.

15 minutes prior to serving, add shrimp, green peas, black beans, wine and Tabasco. Taste, and adjust seasonings.

Serve over white or brown rice.

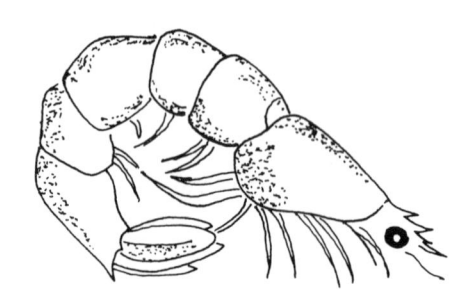

Shrimp Étouffée

Serves 2 (can be doubled)
1.3 grams per serving

1 onion, chopped
½ rib celery, chopped or 1 tsp celery seed
1 green pepper, chopped
2 cloves garlic, minced
1 can tomato paste
water
1 tsp Creole or Cajun seasoning
salt and pepper, to taste
1 lb. raw shrimp, peeled and deveined

Heat oil. Combine onions, celery, green pepper and garlic in large non-stick sauté pan. Cook until vegetables are wilted. Stir tomato paste into vegetable mixture. Add water (up to a cup) until a thick sauce is formed. Season with Creole or Cajun seasoning and salt and pepper. Cover, and simmer on low heat for a total cooking time of 30 minutes, adding shrimp 15 minutes before cooking time is completed.

Serve with rice.

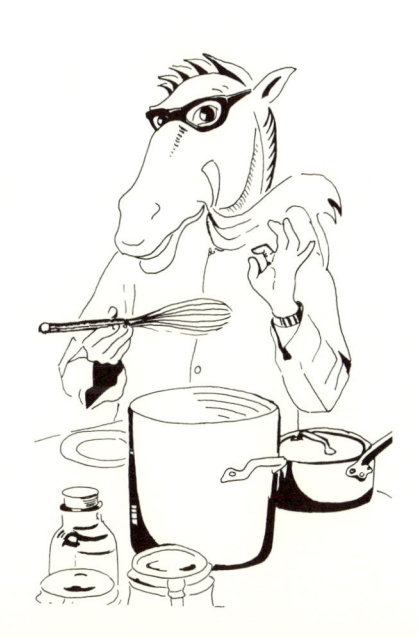

Salmon Croquettes

Serves 4
4.5 grams per serving

Homemade version:

1¼ lb. russet potatoes (4 medium)
2 6-oz salmon steaks
1 Tbs horseradish (optional)
¼ cup chopped scallions
1 Tbs parsley
½ tsp salt, or to taste, and pepper
2 egg whites, beaten
2 tsp butter or margarine
cooking spray

1. Peel and boil potatoes until cooked. Put potatoes through a ricer or Mouli. Bake or microwave salmon until cooked. Remove skin and bones.

2. In a bowl add the salmon, potatoes, horseradish, scallions, parsley, salt and pepper. Mix well. Separately beat the egg whites until frothy. Add the egg whites to the salmon mixture, blending well. Using your hands, take one-eighth of the mixture and form into a ball. Flatten into a burger-sized patty. Repeat with remaining mixture.

3. Spray a large frying pan with cooking spray, and add 1 tsp butter. Cook until browned on one side, using moderate heat. Flip the croquettes and add the other teaspoon of butter. Continue frying until browned.

Quick version: To prepare, proceed as for # 2 and 3 above.

1 7½-oz can salmon
2 cups mashed potato flakes prepared according to package instructions, omitting butter or margarine and substituting skim milk for whole milk
1 Tbs horseradish (optional)
¼ cup chopped scallions
1 Tbs parsley
2 egg whites, beaten
cooking spray, butter

Baked Fish

Serves 4
1.5 grams per serving

Couldn't be simpler.

    4 6-oz (or 1 ½ lbs) fillets of sole, or other fish
    salt, to taste, and pepper
    ¾ cup dry Vermouth
    ¼ cup water
    sliced lemon

Preheat oven to 350°. Spray a baking dish with cooking spray. Salt and pepper the fish, then arrange it in the dish. Pour the Vermouth and water over the fish. Bake for 15 minutes, or until fork flaky. Garnish with sliced lemon.

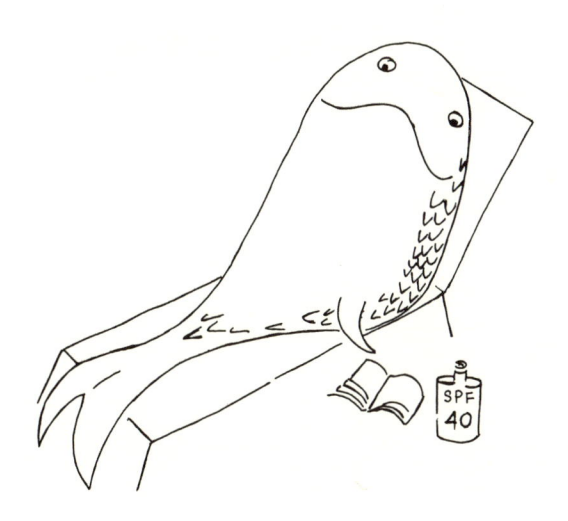

Beef Ball Curry

Serves 4
8 grams per serving

A dish that hits all the right buttons—low-fat, spicy, and something different. Just stuff the meat balls in their tangy sauce into pita pockets.

> 1 lb. lean ground round
> 1 egg, lightly beaten
> ¼ cup bread crumbs
> 1 tsp salt
> ¼ tsp each ground pepper, ground ginger
> 1 tsp Worcestershire sauce
> cooking spray
> 1 large onion, chopped
> 1 cloves garlic, minced or pressed
> 2 Tbs curry powder
> 1 16-oz can tomatoes, diced in medium chunks
> 1 apple, cored and diced
> 1 cup green peas

Combine the ground beef, egg, bread crumbs, salt, pepper, ground ginger and Worcestershire sauce. Shape into small balls. Spray a non-stick skillet with cooking spray and brown the meat balls over medium heat. Lift out and set aside.

Add the onion, garlic and curry powder to the skillet. Cook in the drippings until onion is limp, adding 1 Tbs water, if necessary. Stir in the tomatoes, add their liquid and the apple. Return meat balls to the pan. Add the peas. Cover, and simmer 5-10 minutes until the meatballs are cooked through.

Stuff into pita pockets.

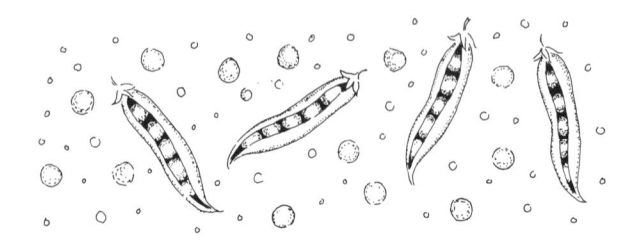

Same Day Sauerbrauten

Serves 6
10 grams per serving

This unique recipe takes only minutes to prepare and has all the flavors of a traditional sauerbraten without the traditional week-long marination.

 ¼ cup flour
 1 tsp salt
 1 tsp ground ginger
 ½ tsp ground allspice
 ½ tsp ground cloves
 ¼ tsp pepper
 2 lbs. lean round steak, trimmed of fat, cut into 1" cubes
 1 Tbs oil
 1 8-oz can tomato sauce
 ¾ cup water
 ½ cup red wine
 ¼ cup cider vinegar
 2 onions, sliced
 2 Tbs sugar (optional)
 1 bay leaf

Place the flour, salt, ginger, allspice, cloves and pepper into a 1-gallon plastic bag. Secure with a twist tie and shake well to blend the ingredients.

Put the cubed beef in the bag and shake to coat the beef. Add oil to a large non-stick skillet and brown the beef on all sides.

Add remaining ingredients to a Dutch oven or suitable pot and cover. Cook the sauerbraten for 1½ to 2 hours, until tender. Thicken with more flour, if necessary, for gravy. Serve over noodles.

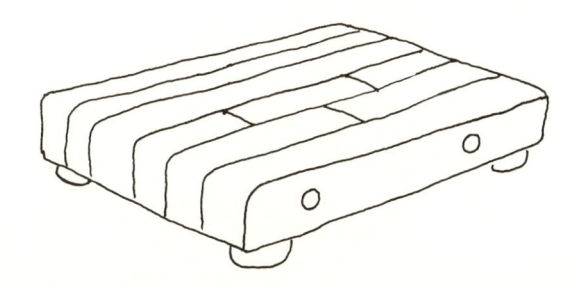

Sweet and Sour Pork

Serves 4
8.5 grams per serving

A low-fat version of the restaurant variety.

    1 lb. pork tenderloin, cubed
    2 tsp oil

    Sauce:
    ¼ cup cold water
    ½ cup sugar
    2 Tbs cornstarch
    1 8-oz can crushed pineapple
    ½ cup green pepper, chopped
    ½ cup red pepper, chopped
    ½ cup cider vinegar
    ½ cup catsup
    1 clove garlic, minced
    ¼ tsp powdered ginger
    2 Tbs low sodium soy sauce
    Tabasco, to taste

Heat the oil in a non-stick skillet. Add the pork and brown evenly on all sides. Reduce heat, cover, and simmer until cooked through.

Meanwhile, in a 1-quart sauce pan, stir together the water, sugar, and cornstarch. Bring to a boil, then reduce heat. Add the remaining ingredients, stirring constantly until thick. Add sauce to the pork, stir and heat through.

Serve with rice.

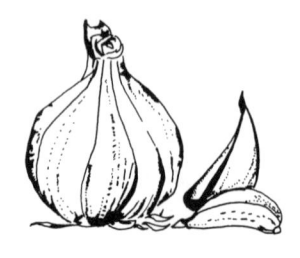

Skillet Pork and Cabbage

Serves 4
6 grams per serving

1 tsp oil
1 pound butterflied pork, trimmed of all visible fat
2 tsp water
salt, to taste and pepper
2 whole cloves
1 bay leaf
1 medium head cabbage, sliced thinly
2 tart apples, diced
1 medium onion, chopped
¼ cup sugar
1½ tsp all-purpose flour
2 tsp water
2 tsp vinegar
salt and pepper, to taste

Heat oil in a skillet. Brown the pork on both sides. Add 2 tsps water, salt, cloves and bay leaf. Cover and simmer over low-moderate heat for 20 minutes. Remove the pork, discard cloves and bay leaf. Add the cabbage, apple, and onion. In a bowl, mix together the sugar, flour, water, vinegar, salt and pepper. Pour the mixture over the cabbage. Stir. Cover and simmer the cabbage for 5 minutes. Return pork to the skillet and place over the cabbage. Cover and cook an additional 10 minutes, or until heated through.

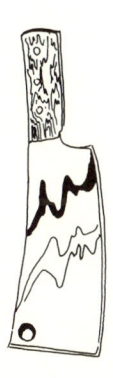

Pizza

Serves 1
9 grams per serving

We have never met anyone who hated pizza, even with spinach on it. At spas everywhere, tortilla-crust pizza is served as a treat. This recipe, and all its variations, can be served for lunch or dinner, any day of the week. But don't even contemplate pepperoni!

The basic recipe is for one serving. But by expanding the ingredients you can have lots of these pizzas flying out of the oven. There is no law that pizza has to be made with mozzarella, any good melting cheese is fine. And hard cheeses like asiago and pecorino are particularly tangy.

> 1 9" flour tortilla
> 1 oz shredded cheese (4 generous tablespoons)
> Quick pizza sauce (recipe follows)
> Any combination of vegetables: thin zucchini disks, sliced mushrooms, roasted red peppers, green pepper strips, onion slices, artichoke hearts, etc.

Preheat oven to 350°. Before baking pizza have all ingredients ready. Place tortilla on a pizza pan or baking sheet and warm in the oven for 1 minute. Remove from the oven and spread a thin layer of pizza sauce on the tortilla. Add vegetables of choice, and sprinkle grated cheese over pizza. Place in oven, but keep an eye on the pizza, the rim of the thin crust will brown quickly.

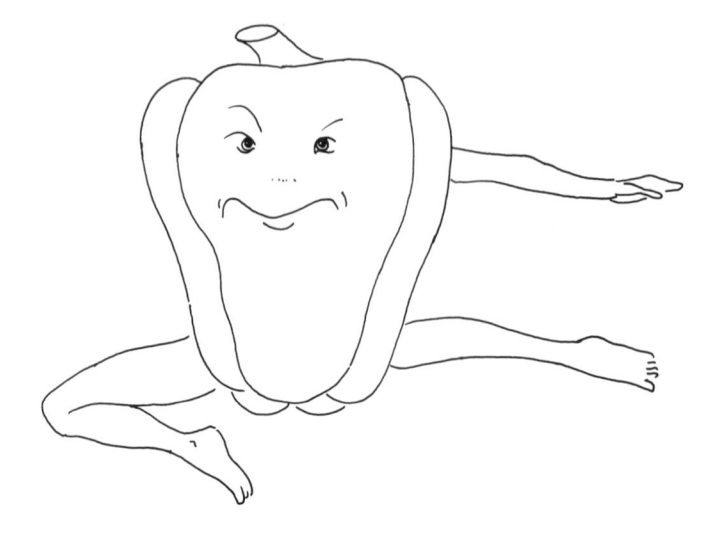

Quick Pizza Sauce

Makes approx. 2 cups
0 grams per ¼ cup

1 6-oz can tomato paste
1 cup water
½ tsp sugar
¼ tsp salt
1 Tbs Italian seasoning
1 garlic clove, minced
1 Tbs red wine or 1 tsp balsamic vinegar (optional)

Put all ingredients in a sauce pan and stir well. Simmer on low heat for 10-15 minutes. Refrigerate unused portion for up to a week. Or freeze in individual portions for up to three months.

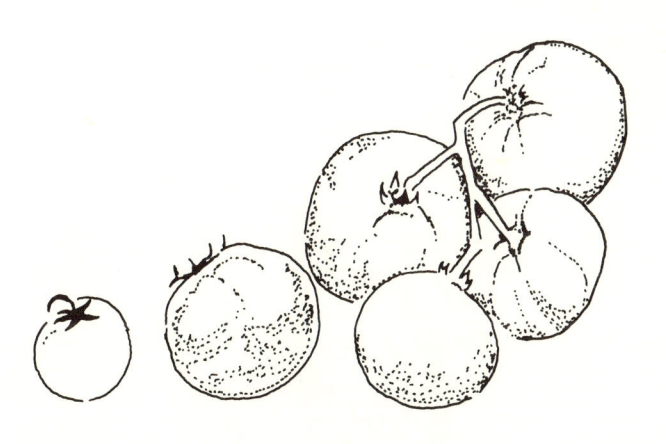

Vegetarian Chili

Serves 8
1.7 grams per serving

Best made in a crock pot. If you cook the chili on the range, be sure to stir the pot every once in a while to keep the chili from sticking. This chili also makes a great bean burrito. Place chili in center of tortilla, dollop with sour half & half, salsa and chopped scallion. Roll up and serve.

- 1 6-oz can tomato paste
- 1 can beer
- 1 15- or 16-oz can diced tomatoes (use liquid)
- 1 16-oz can dark red kidney beans
- 2 16-oz cans small red beans
- 1 pkg. (box) frozen small lima beans (or 1 cup from bag)
- 3 cloves garlic, pressed or minced
- 1 large onion, diced
- 1 green bell pepper, diced
- 2-3 Tbs chili powder*
- 1 Tbs ground cumin
- 1 Tbs oregano
- 1 Tbs Tabasco, or to taste

Put all of the above ingredients in a crock pot. Stir well. If not enough liquid, add water. Cook for approximately 3 hours. Check seasoning. At the end of the cooking period, add 1 tsp (or less) salt and other spices, if needed.

* Some commercial chili powders contain oregano, cumin and garlic. If you can't find pure chili powder, adjust seasonings.

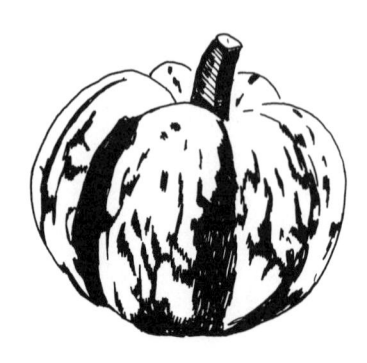

SWEETS

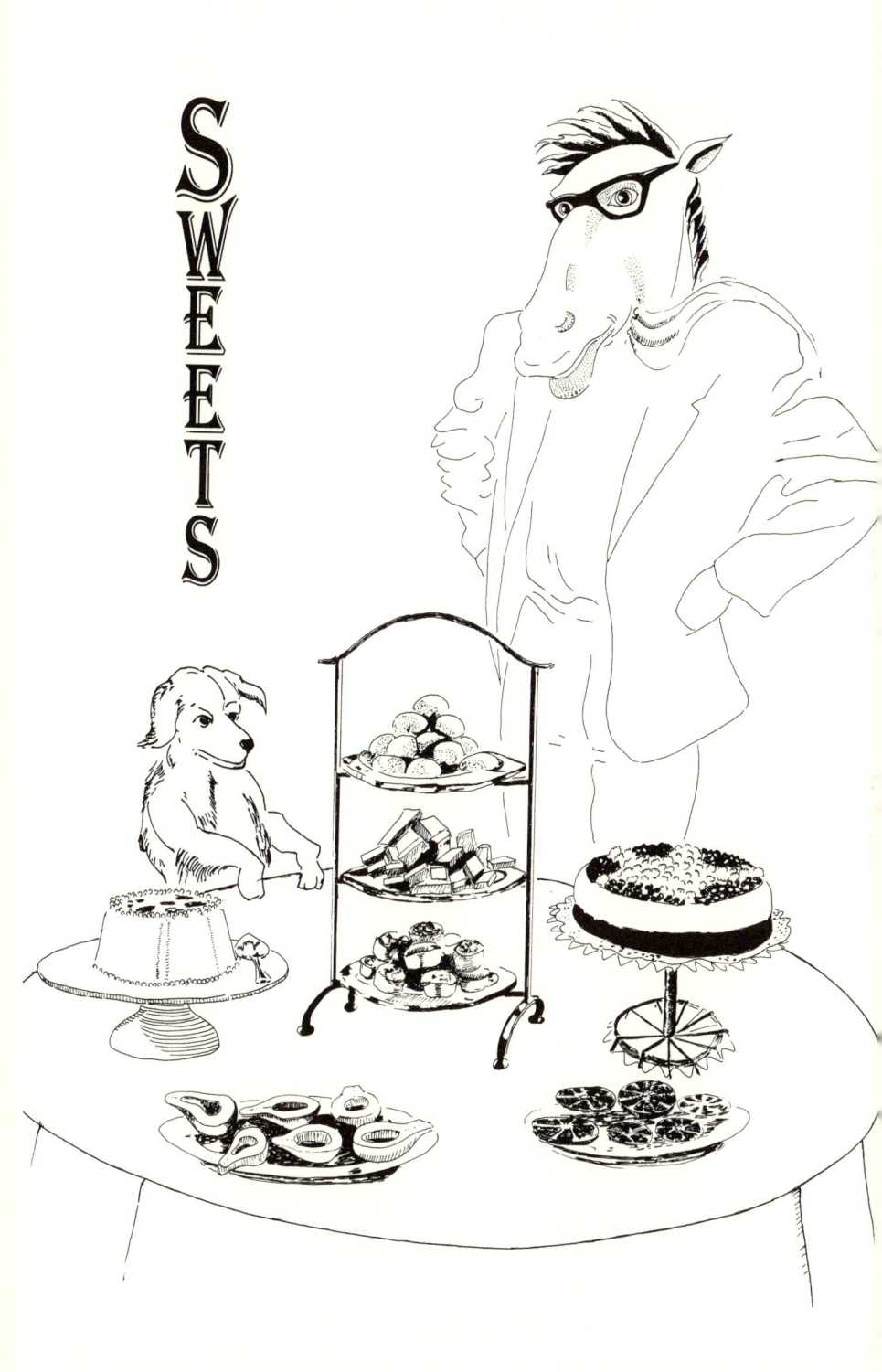

Pavlova Pie

Serves 8
0 grams per serving

Fill this puffy pie shell with sherbet, sorbet or frozen yogurt. Top with berries, sliced bananas, peaches or other fruit in season.

>   3 fresh egg whites
>   scant ½ tsp lemon juice
>   ¼ tsp cream of tartar
>   ½ cup powdered sugar
>   ½ tsp vanilla extract
>   cooking spray

Preheat oven to 275°. Put the egg whites, lemon juice and cream of tartar in a large mixing bowl. Beat the mixture with an electric mixer until very frothy. Gradually add sugar and continue beating until stiff peaks form. Add vanilla and beat for 1 minute more.

Spray a 9" pie pan with cooking spray. With a spatula, spoon the meringue into the pie plate, taking care to build up the sides into a nest.

Bake the Pavlova for 1 hour, then reduce heat to 250° and bake for another 30 minutes. Pavlova should be dry and crisp, but not brown.

Cool Pavlova. If making ahead, store in a moisture-proof container. Prior to serving, spoon frozen yogurt, sorbet or sherbet evenly into pie shell. Top with berries or fruit.

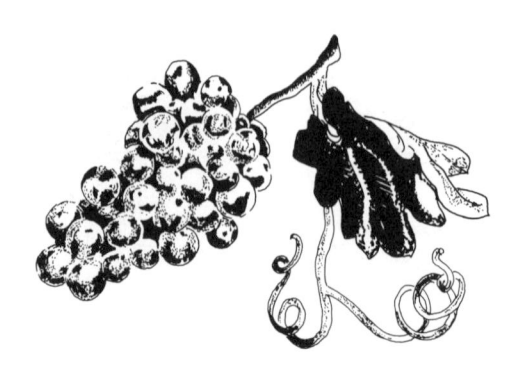

Pepper Cookies

Makes 16 cookies
0.4 gram per cookie

Yep, it's true, folks, each cookie contains less than half a gram of fat. Spice cookies are nice any time of year, but these are particularly welcome around the holidays when temptation comes knocking.

    1 egg
    ½ cup sugar
    1 cup flour
    ¼ tsp each: salt, ground white pepper, cloves, nutmeg, ginger
    ½ tsp cinnamon
    ½ tsp baking powder
    1 lemon peel, finely grated (yellow skin only)
    1 Tbs water
    powdered sugar

Whisk egg and sugar in a small bowl until light and fluffy. Sift flour and spices together in a medium bowl. Add grated lemon peel.

Add the sugar-egg mixture to the flour-spice mixture, stirring with a spoon. Add the water, and with your hands form the dough into a ball. Wrap the ball in plastic wrap and chill for 1 hour.

Preheat oven to 350°. Spray a baking sheet with cooking spray. Flour your hands for smooth handling of the batter, and form into 16 small balls. Bake for 20 minutes.

Cool on a rack. When cool enough to handle, roll each cookie in powdered sugar.

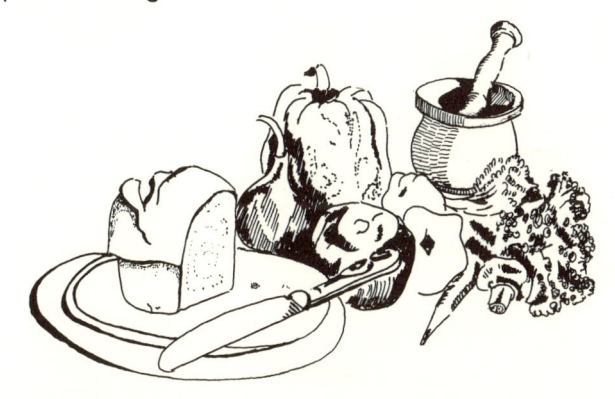

Librada's Floating Island

Serves 6-8
0 grams per serving

This variation of the famous floating island dessert is surrounded by a sea of gooey caramel. Caramel syrup boiled in the microwave oven is surprisingly easy to make. If you've been daunted in the past by burnt caramel, or syrup that wouldn't caramelize, try the never-fail microwave method below.

> ½ cup sugar for caramel sauce
> ½ cup water
> 8 fresh egg whites
> ½ cup sugar for floating island

Place the sugar and water in a 1-pt Pyrex measuring cup. Stir well. Microwave at high for 9 minutes. At this point the water and sugar should be boiling furiously, but will still be clear in color.

Start timing in 1-minute increments: Set the microwave on high for 1 minute, keeping an eye on the color of the caramel. It will begin to turn light amber. Set the microwave on high for 1 minute more, it will turn a honey color. When the caramel looks like honey it's done. Turn off the microwave and remove carefully—the syrup will be *very* hot.

Immediately pour the caramel into a bundt pan and rotate to coat the sides. The caramel will harden very quickly.

Preheat the oven to 350°. Fill a large shallow baking pan with 1 inch of water and place the pan on the middle oven rack.

In a large, clean bowl, using the whisk attachment of an electric mixer, beat the egg whites with the sugar for 20 minutes.

Spoon the meringue into the bundt pan with the caramel. Rap the pan sharply a couple of times to burst any large bubbles in the pan. Bake the meringue for 30-35 minutes, or until just set. Remove from the oven and from the water bath. Carefully, loosen the meringue around the edges and when cool, invert onto a large colorful plate.

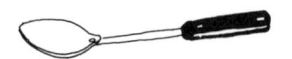

Low Fat Flan

Serves 6
1.5 grams per serving

Only 100 calories! Use the method on the previous page for making caramel syrup.

 ½ cup sugar
 ½ cup water
 2 cups 1% milk
 1 egg
 2 egg whites
 2½ Tbs sugar
 ½ tsp vanilla extract
 1 tsp grated lemon or orange rind

Prepare caramel syrup according to instructions on previous page. Pour the syrup equally into 6 custard cups.

Preheat oven to 325°. Scald milk in a medium saucepan. In a bowl, whisk together the eggs and egg whites with 2½ Tbs sugar. Add the milk to the bowl slowly, whisking constantly. Add vanilla and lemon or orange rind.

Pour custard mixture into prepared cups. Place custard cups in a deep pan. Pour 1 inch hot water in the pan. Bake the custard for 40–45 minutes. To test for doneness, insert a knife near the edge of the cup, if the blade comes out clean, the custard is cooked through.

Remove flan from oven and refrigerate until very cold. To serve, run a knife around the edges of the cups. Turn upside-down on dessert plates. The caramel will form a sauce around the custard.

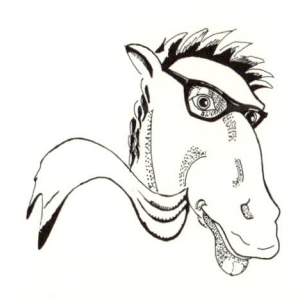

Dannon Brownies

Makes 16 brownies
1 gram per brownie

It's hard to improve on these brownies that were developed by the Dannon yogurt people. Prepared with egg whites and yogurt, the fat savings are a whopping 72 grams.

    1 pkg. Brownie mix
    1/3 cup nonfat yogurt
    1 tsp vanilla
    2 egg whites

Preheat oven to 350°. Combine brownie mix, yogurt, vanilla and egg whites in a medium bowl. Mix well. The batter will be thick. Spread in a 9" x 13" baking pan and bake for 22 to 24 minutes. Or bake 32 minutes in a 9" x 9" pan. Cool before cutting.

Tip: When using a glass pan, lower oven temperature to 325°.

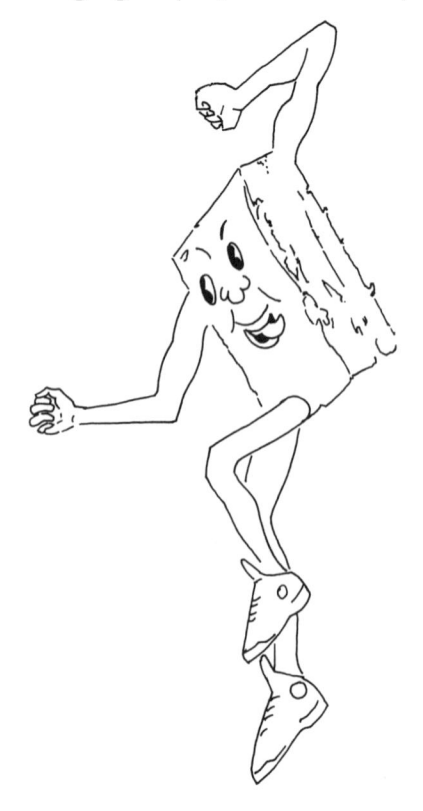

Oranges in Wine

Serves 4
0 grams per serving

Nice when served with coconut kisses.

    4 oranges
    ¼ cup powdered sugar
    1 cup dry red wine
    1 stick cinnamon
    ¼ tsp freshly-ground nutmeg

Peel and seed oranges. Slice oranges in ¼" rounds and place in a small bowl. Sprinkle with confectioner's sugar. Add the wine, cinnamon and nutmeg. Serve very cold.

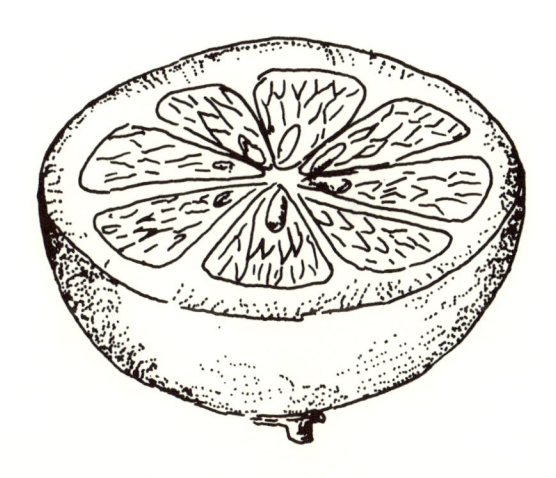

Coconut Kisses

Makes 48 kisses
3 grams per 6 kisses

3 egg whites
¼ tsp salt
1 cup sugar
1 tsp vanilla
1 cup flaked, shredded coconut

Preheat oven to 300°. With an electric mixer, beat egg whites and salt until stiff peaks form. Very slowly add the sugar, continuing to beat the mixture. Use a spatula to gently fold in vanilla and coconut.

Drop the batter from a teaspoon onto a greased and floured cookie sheet. Bake for about 30 minutes. Keep an eye on them during the last cooking minutes—don't allow your kisses to get singed.

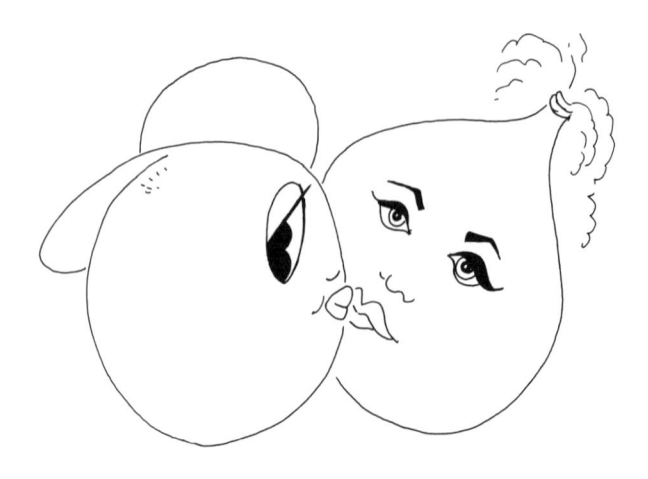

Baked Apples

Serves 4
0 grams per serving

Zeb's favorite way to eat apples.

    4 Rome beauty apples,
    4-6 Tbs pure maple syrup
    4 Tbs golden raisins

Preheat oven to 350°. Wash and core the apples, creating a reservoir for the filling and taking care to leave a ½ inch base. Place the apples in an oven-proof baking pan and cover the bottom of the pan with ½ inch of water. Divide the raisins and place equal amounts in the reservoirs. Fill, but don't overfill the reservoirs with maple syrup. Bake for 45 minutes. Serve cold or at room temperature.

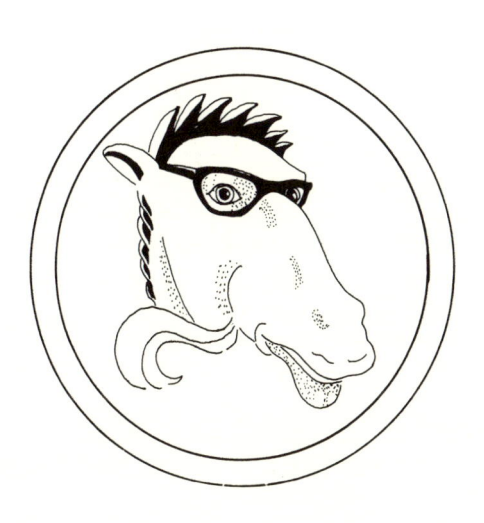

Almond Biscotti

Makes 48 biscotti
2 grams per biscotti

There are several compelling reasons why you should bake your own biscotti, not the least of which is cost. A dozen biscotti from a bakery can cost over $10. These biscotti are easy to make, and the preparation time runs only about 20 minutes. Our favorite dunking cookies!

- ¾ cup shelled almonds
- 2 cups white flour
- 1 cup sugar
- 1 tsp baking powder
- ¼ tsp salt
- 4 Tbs butter, melted
- 2 large eggs, lightly beaten
- 1 tsp vanilla extract

Preheat oven to 325°. Toast the almonds on a baking sheet for 5 minutes. When cool, measure ¼ cup of the nuts and grind them finely. Combine and stir together the dry ingredients except the almonds in a large mixing bowl.

In a small bowl, combine the melted butter, eggs and vanilla, beating lightly. Add the liquid ingredients to the dry ingredients and stir until well-blended. Add both the ground and whole nuts.

Knead the dough until the mixture is smooth. Shape the dough into two 12" logs. Wrap in plastic wrap and flatten each log to ¾ inch thickness. Refrigerate for at least ½ hour.

Heat oven to 325°. Unwrap logs and bake on a baking sheet for 30 minutes, or until a toothpick inserted in the center comes out clean.

Cool logs on a wire rack for 10 minutes. Using a serrated knife, slice the logs diagonally ½" thick.

Reduce heat to 275°. Stand the biscotti upright on the baking sheet and return to oven. Bake the biscotti for 30 minutes, until lightly toasted. Cool on wire racks.

Chocolate Angel Cake

Serves 8
1.6 grams per serving

A transport to Heaven for chocolate lovers. If, like Zeb, you hate to waste food, beat the egg yolks together with a little water, put in a bowl and microwave on medium for 2 minutes. Top your dog's food with a portion of the scrambled yolks. Unlike humans, dogs do not convert fat to cholesterol. If you don't have a dog get one—studies show dog owners live longer.

1 cup cake flour
¼ cup unsweetened cocoa
1½ cups sugar
10-12 egg whites (or 1¼ cups), room temperature
¼ tsp salt
1½ tsps cream of tartar
1 tsp vanilla (or ½ tsp vanilla and ½ tsp almond extract)

Preheat oven to 350°. Sift flour, cocoa and ¾ cup sugar together 3 times. In a large mixing bowl, combine egg whites, salt, cream of tartar and the extract(s). Beat at high speed with an electric mixer until foamy. Gradually add the remaining ¾ cup sugar continuing to beat until whites form stiff peaks.

Sift ¼ of the flour mixture over the egg whites and fold into the batter with a spatula. Repeat with remaining flour mixture, taking care not to overfold as this will deflate the batter.

Place the batter in an ungreased 10" tube pan. Run a knife through the batter to remove air pockets. Bake for 40-45 minutes.

Turn the tube pan upside down onto an inverted funnel and cool the cake for at least an hour. When cool, run a knife around the edges and remove from pan.

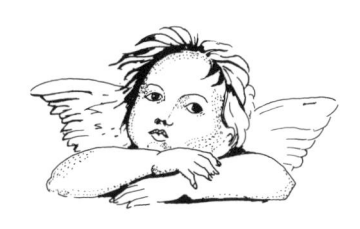

Chocolate Mint Meltaways

Makes 24 puffs
2.3 grams per puff

This a serious recipe. You'll be in serious trouble if you remove the puffs from the oven prematurely! Try this recipe with Butterscotch morsels instead of chocolate mint. Fat gram counts are based on using Nestlé morsels. Other brands may contain up to one-third more fat.

   3 egg whites
   2/3 cup sugar
   1 cup (7 ounces) chocolate mint morsels
   cooking spray

Beat egg whites with an electric mixture on high speed until peaks form. Gradually add the sugar until whites are stiff and glossy. Fold in mint chocolate morsels.

Heat oven to 375°. Spray a baking sheet with cooking spray. Drop puffs by teaspoonfuls onto the baking sheet. Place in oven. Immediately turn off heat. Leave the puffs in the oven overnight or for 8 hours. Do not open oven.

Store in an air-tight container. The puffs will keep up to a week.

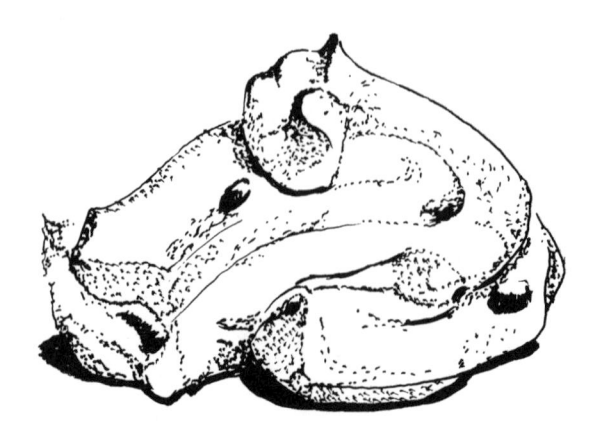

Poached Pears

Serves 6
0 gram per serving

A perfect finale to a low fat dinner. And as a dinner party bonus, you can make this the day before and serve it cold. Save time by poaching the pears in the microwave.

- 1½ cups red wine or port
- 1 cup sugar
- 2 Tbs fresh lemon juice
- 1 cinnamon stick
- 6 whole cloves
- Couple grinds black pepper
- 6 ripe but firm Bosc or Bartlett pears

Preheat oven to 350°. In an enamel or other non-reactive saucepan, bring the wine or port and sugar to a boil. Add 1 Tbs lemon juice, cinnamon stick, cloves, and a dusting of black pepper.

Using a vegetable peeler, peel the pears. Cut in half lengthwise and core. (A melon baller does a very neat job.) Immerse the pears in cold water with the remaining 1 Tbs lemon juice while the syrup cooks for another 5 minutes.

Arrange the pears snugly in a baking dish. Pour the syrup over the pears. Cover with foil and bake for 30-45 minutes, depending on ripeness of pears. Pears are ready when a toothpick glides in easily.

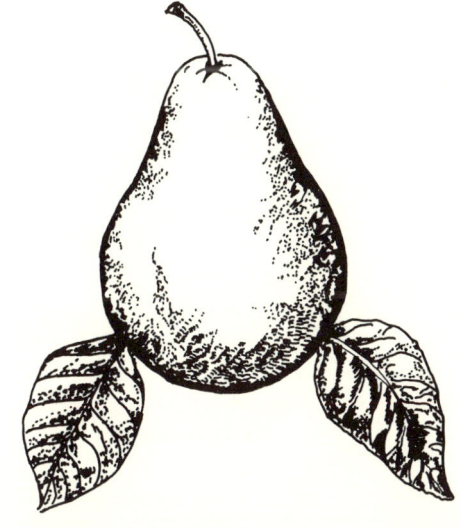

No Fat (No Kidding) Pie Crust

Makes one 9" pie crust
0 grams per serving

Use your favorite pie filling in this easy-to-prepare crust.

- 1 cup Grape Nuts
- ½ cup apple juice concentrate
- ½ tsp cinnamon

Preheat oven to 375°. Mix ingredients in a pie pan. Press into pan and bake for 8-10 minutes.

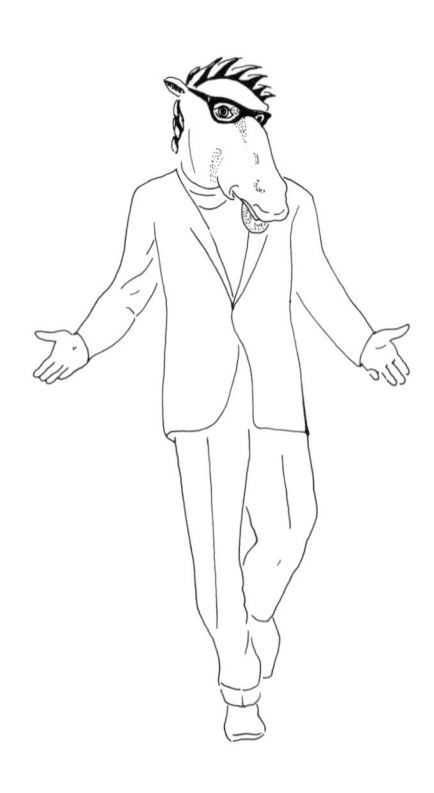

Pretty Peaches

Serves 4
0 grams per serving

If you have parfait glasses, dust them off for this recipe. If not, any attractive glassware may be used to present the colorful layers of this dessert. Canned peaches may be substituted for fresh.

  2 cups fresh or frozen raspberries
  ½ cup orange juice
  1 cup nonfat yogurt (vanilla flavored works well)
  2 Tbs orange marmalade
  4 large ripe peaches
  mint leaves, for garnish (optional)

Mix orange juice and raspberries in a bowl, cover and refrigerate for several hours until well-chilled. In another bowl mix the yogurt and marmalade. Cover and chill.

Peel, pit and slice the fresh peaches. If using canned, drain syrup.

On the bottom of a parfait glass, spoon one-eighth of the raspberry mixture. Add a layer of sliced peaches. Then spoon ¼ portion of yogurt-marmalade mixture on peaches. Arrange the remaining peaches over the yogurt and top with the remaining raspberry mixture. Garnish with sprigs of mint.

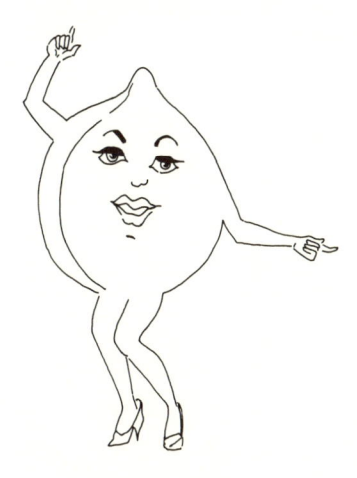

Frozen Lemon Crunch

Serves 6
4 grams per serving

This is a terrific recipe as is, but for a glamorous presentation process the crunch in an ice-cream maker (omitting the topping), spoon into a Pavlova shell (recipe on page 154) and top with the corn flake mix.

  1 cup evaporated skim milk
  ¼ cup + 1 Tbs fresh lemon juice
  2 large egg whites
  ½ cup sugar
  ½ tsp salt
  1 Tbs grated lemon rind
  2 drops yellow food coloring (optional)
  ½ cup finely-crushed corn flakes
  2 Tbs butter, melted
  1 Tbs sugar

Freeze the evaporated milk in a small bowl until soft ice crystals form around the edges of the bowl, about 15-20 minutes. With an electric beater, whip until stiff and return bowl to freezer. In a medium bowl, add the lemon juice, egg whites, sugar and salt and beat until thick and creamy. Add the lemon rind and food coloring, if desired.

Fold in the whipped milk and put in a 8½ x 4½ x 2¾" loaf pan. Return the mixture to the freezer. Meanwhile, mix corn flakes, butter and 1 Tbs sugar in a bowl. Sprinkle mixture over top of pan and freeze until firm (about 2 hours).

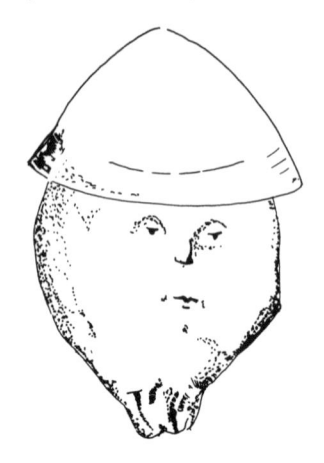

Chocolate Cupcakes with Mint Glaze

Makes 8
5 grams per serving

Cupcakes:
1 ½ cups flour
1 cup sugar
3 Tbs unsweetened cocoa powder
½ tsp salt
3 Tbs butter, softened
1 Tbs pure vanilla
1 Tbs white vinegar
1 cup cold water

Mint Glaze:
¾ cup powdered sugar
¼ tsp mint extract
about 1 Tbs milk

Preheat oven to 350°. Line cupcake tin with eight paper liners. Sift dry ingredients together in a medium bowl. Add remaining ingredients, mixing well.

Pour batter into prepared tin, evenly distributing batter. Bake cupcakes for 30–35 minutes, or until cupcakes spring back when lightly touched. Cool on a rack. To make glaze, stir powdered sugar, mint extract and milk together until well-blended. Use enough milk to make mixture of drizzling consistency. While cupcakes are still warm, drizzle with glaze.

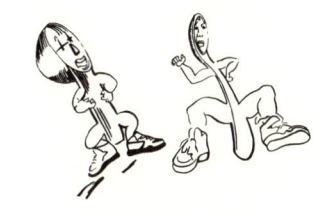

Orange Sponge Cake

Serves 12
1 gram per serving

Tah Dah! The perfect cake to end this low-fat odyssey. An adaptation of this recipe appeared in *Ladies' Home Journal* in January, 1993.

>   1½ cups all-purpose flour
>   1¼ tsp baking powder
>   ¼ tsp salt
>   3 large eggs, separated
>   1 cup sugar, divided
>   2 tsp hot water
>   ½ cup fresh orange juice
>   1 tsp vanilla
>   1 tsp grated orange peel
>   3 egg whites

Preheat oven to 350°. In a large bowl, sift together flour, baking powder and salt.

Beat egg yolks, ¾ cup sugar and hot water in a mixer bowl at medium speed until the mixture is light and swirls up when the beaters are lifted. Add orange juice and continue beating at low speed until well blended. Beat in vanilla and orange peel for 2 minutes. In 3 batches, gently fold the orange, egg, and sugar mixture into the dry ingredients. Do not overstir.

Wash and dry the mixer bowl and beaters. Beat all 6 egg whites at medium speed until frothy. Add the remaining sugar and increase beater speed to high. Whisk one-third of the beaten whites into the batter, then fold in the remaining whites. Spoon batter into an ungreased tube pan.

Bake the cake for approximately 30 minutes, until it springs back when lightly touched. Turn the tube pan upside down onto an inverted funnel and cool the cake for at least an hour. When cool, run a knife around the edges and remove from pan.

APPENDIX

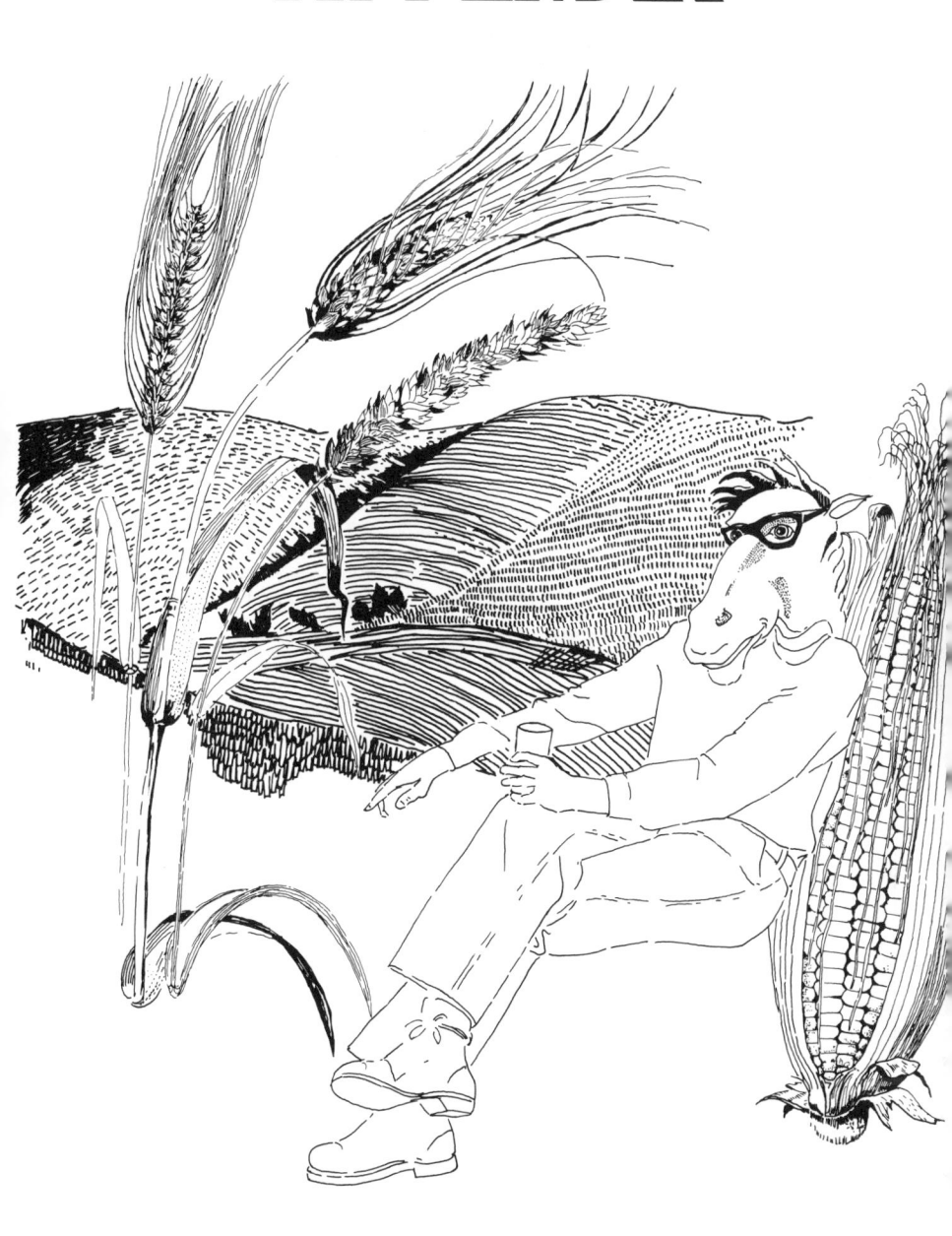

A Month of Great Low-Fat Menus

10 Grams and Under

✶= An Eat Like a Horse Recipe

BREAKFAST
✶Raisin Bread with ✶Apple Butter

LUNCH
✶Escarole Soup
Nonfat Breadsticks

SNACK
Rice cakes with ✶Apple Butter

DINNER
✶Baked fish
Microwaved Sweet Potato with ✶Jalapeño Jelly
✶Corn Pudding

DESSERT
✶Chocolate Angel Cake

Total Fat: 9.4 grams

BREAKFAST
✶Breakfast Cake

LUNCH
Tuna or Turkey Breast pita Sandwich with Veggies, Sprouts and Salsa

SNACK
Fruit Smoothie

DINNER
✶Salmon Croquettes
✶Stewed Tomatoes

DESSERT
✶Orange Sponge Cake

Total Fat: 10 grams

BREAKFAST
*Popover with Jam
*Yogurt with Fruit

LUNCH
*Curried Broccoli Soup
Fat-free Crackers

SNACK
*Nutty Beans

DINNER
*Honey Mustard Chicken
Rice
*Stir-fried Pea pods

DESSERT
*Pretty Peaches

Total Fat: 8.5 grams

BREAKFAST
*Granola with Fruit

LUNCH
Tossed Salad: Greens, Veggies, Sprouts with ¼ cup *Blue Cheese Dressing

SNACK
*Stuffed Cherry Tomatoes

DINNER
*Turkey and Rice Pepper Boats

DESSERT
*Baked Apples

Total Fat: 9.4 grams

BREAKFAST
*Raisin Bread

LUNCH
*Potato Onion Pie
(Microwaved leftover)
Steamed Veggies

SNACK
*Roquefort 'Shrooms

DINNER
*Tuna Creole
Green Salad with *Caesar dressing

DESSERT
*Pretty Peaches

Total Fat: 8.5 grams

BREAKFAST
*Blueberry Muffin

LUNCH
*Pepper Cream Soup
2 oz Sliced Turkey Breast on Rye Bread

SNACK
Rice Cakes with *Apple Butter

DINNER
*Spinach Fettuccine with Lemon Ricotta Sauce
Steamed Veggies

DESSERT
*Oranges in Wine
*Coconut Kisses

Total Fat: 9.3 grams

BREAKFAST
Cereal with skim milk and fresh fruit

LUNCH
*Vegetarian Chili Burrito

SNACK
Fat free crackers

DINNER
*Shrimp Fiesta
*Baked Artichokes

DESSERT
*2 Pepper Cookies

Total Fat: 10 grams

BREAKFAST
*Bran Muffin

LUNCH
*Lentil & Brown Rice Soup

SNACK
*Oven-roasted corn chips with *Mock Guac

DINNER
*Chili Blanco
*Yellow Squash

DESSERT
*Floating Island

Total Fat: 9.7 grams

BREAKFAST
*Microwave Oatmeal

LUNCH
*Macaroni, Bean, and Spinach Soup
Italian Bread with *Roasted Garlic

SNACK
*Ragin' Cajun Popcorn

DINNER
*Shrimp Étouffée with Rice
Steamed Spinach

DESSERT
*Dannon Brownie

Total Fat: 8.5 grams

BREAKFAST
*Granola with Skim milk and Fresh Fruit

LUNCH
*Tuna Pasta Salad

SNACK
Fruit Smoothie

DINNER
*Cheese and Chicken Enchiladas
*Black Bean Salad

DESSERT
*Poached Pears

Total Fat: 9.6 grams

20 Grams and Under

BREAKFAST
Fat-free Cereal with skim milk and fruit

LUNCH
✻Rigatoni with Mushrooms
(Microwaved Leftover)

SNACK
¼ cup ✻Jalapeño Dip
with ✻Oven-Crisped Corn Chips

DINNER
✻Chicken Cutlets with Rice
✻Spinach Soufflé

DESSERT
Apple Pie Made with ✻Fat-free Pie Crust

Total Fat: 17.6 grams

BREAKFAST
✻Blueberry muffin and fresh fruit

LUNCH
✻Twice-baked Potato
(Microwaved leftover)
Green Salad with ✻Ranch Dressing

SNACK
Fruit Smoothie

DINNER
✻Sweet and Sour Cabbage
1 slice rye bread

DESSERT
2 ✻Mint Meltaways

Total Fat: 19.4 grams

BREAKFAST
✻Granola with ✻Yogurt and Fruit

LUNCH
✻Shredded Carrot Salad
Tuna in pita Stuffed with Sprouts

SNACK
3 ✻Cannellini Rollups

DINNER
✻Gnocchi with Pork
Green Salad with any no-fat dressing

DESSERT
✻Chocolate Angel Cake

Total Fat: 17.3 grams

BREAKFAST
Poached Egg on Toast

LUNCH
✻1-2-3 Soup
Green Salad with ✻Adult's Only Dressing

SNACK
Fruit Smoothie

DINNER
✻Money Bags
✻Stir-Fried Pea Pods

DESSERT
✻Pavlova Pie

Total Fat: 17.5

20 Grams and Under

BREAKFAST
✳Blueberry Muffins

LUNCH
4 ✳Corn Pancakes
Steamed Veggies

SNACK
Fruit Smoothie

DINNER
✳Shells Florentine
Salad with ✳ Caesar Dressing

DESSERT
2 ✳Almond Biscotti

Total Fat: 17.4 grams

BREAKFAST
✳Breakfast Cake

LUNCH
2 oz Smoked Turkey, ✳Corn Relish
on 2 Slices Bread

SNACK
✳Ragin' Cajun Popcorn

DINNER
✳Rosemary Roasted Potatoes
✳Oven Baked Chicken
✳Spinach and Egg

DESSERT
✳Baked Apples

Total Fat: 18 grams

BREAKFAST
✳Raisin Bread with ✳Apple Butter

LUNCH
✳Tubetti in Ricotta Pepper Sauce
Mixed green salad with fat-free dressing

SNACK
Fruit Smoothie

DINNER
✳Eat Like a Horse Chicken
✳Rosemary Roasted Potatoes
✳Hungarian Green Beans

DESSERT
Any under 6 grams

Total Fat: 19.2 grams

BREAKFAST
✳2 Bran Muffins

LUNCH
Lean Cold Cuts on Rye with Mustard

SNACK
Julienned Veggies with ✳Frijomole
(¼ cup)

DINNER
✳Turkey Tetrazzini

DESSERT
1 slice store-bought fat-free Cake

Total Fat: 18.2 grams

BREAKFAST
*Southwestern Eggs

LUNCH
*Easy Ratatouille
*Baked Rice
(Microwaved Leftover)

SNACK
Rice Cake with *Apple Butter

DINNER
*Tandoori Chicken with Rice
*Cucumber Raita

DESSERT
*Lemon Crunch

Total Fat: 19.7 grams

BREAKFAST
2 *Bran Muffins

LUNCH
*Greek Lemon soup
1 slice pumpernickel

SNACK
*Tapenade with low-fat crackers

DINNER
*Beef Ball Curry

DESSERT
*Dannon Brownie

Total Fat: 19.5

25 Grams and Under

BREAKFAST
*Breakfast Cake

LUNCH
*Vegetarian Chili Burrito

SNACK
*Herbed Crostini

DINNER
*Chicken Yakitori with Rice
*Cucumber Salad

DESSERT
Any under 10 grams per serving

Total Fat: 24.7 grams

BREAKFAST
2 *Blueberry Muffins

LUNCH
*Chicken & Pork Adobo with Rice
(Microwaved Leftover)

SNACK
Rice Cake with *Apple Butter

DINNER
*Gorgonzola Lasagna
Tossed Salad with fat-free Dressing

DESSERT
3*Chocolate Mint Meltaways

Total Fat: 25 grams

BREAKFAST
*Eggs Sardou

LUNCH
Sliced Turkey Breast in pita
with *Mango Salsa

SNACK
Fruit Smoothie

DINNER
*Pizza

DESSERT
2 *Almond Biscotti

Total Fat: 23.5 grams

BREAKFAST
Poached Egg with Toast

LUNCH
*Shells Florentine
(Microwaved Leftover)
Tossed green salad with fat-free Dressing

SNACK
*Oven-crisped Chips with *Jalapeño Dip

DINNER
*Sweet and Sour Pork with Rice

DESSERT
*Pavlova Pie

Total Fat: 24.5 grams

BREAKFAST
✳Granola with ✳Yogurt and Fruit

LUNCH
✳Gorgonzola Lasagna
(Microwaved Leftover)
Tossed Salad with ✳Buttermilk Dressing

SNACK
✳Tapenade with Crackers

DINNER
✳Sloppy Jalopies
✳Creamy Potato Salad

DESSERT
✳Baked Apples

Total Fat: 22.2 grams

BREAKFAST
✳Southwestern Eggs

LUNCH
✳Librada's Cloud Soup
1 slice French Bread

SNACK
No fat Pretzels

DINNER
✳Adobo with Rice
✳Orange Glazed Carrots

DESSERT
Any under 5 grams

Total Fat: 23 grams

BREAKFAST
✳Microwave Oatmeal with fresh fruit

LUNCH
✳Salmon Pasta Salad

SNACK
Fruit Smoothie

DINNER
✳Same Day Sauerbrauten with Egg Noodles
✳Glazed Brussels Sprouts

DESSERT
✳Frozen Lemon Crunch

Total Fat: 25 grams

BREAKFAST
✳Eggs Sardou

LUNCH
✳Lentil and Brown Rice Soup

SNACK
✳Shrimp-Cucumber Dip with
Celery and Carrot Sticks

DINNER
✳Arroz con Pollo

DESSERT
✳Orange Sponge Cake

Total Fat: 23.5 grams

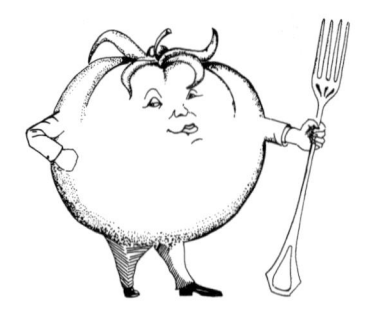

INDEX

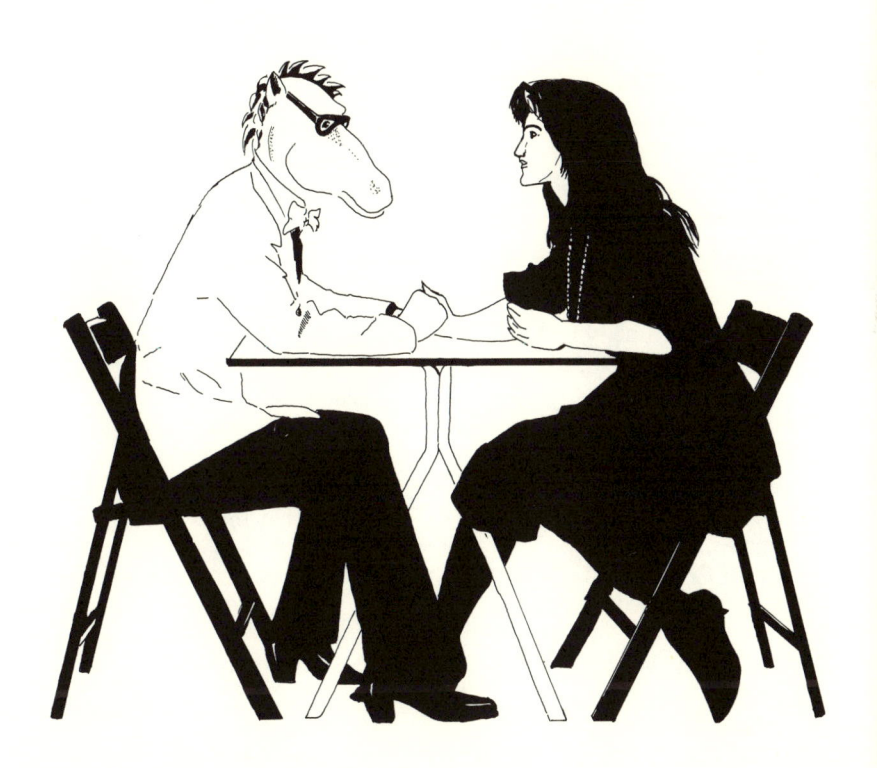

—A—

Angel Cake, Chocolate, 163
Apple Butter, 46
Apples, Baked, 161
Artichokes, Baked, 107
Asparagus, Steamed, 122

—B—

Beef Ball Curry, 146
Biscotti, Almond, 162
Blueberry Muffins, 17
Bran Muffins, 23
Bread, Raisin, 26
Brownies, Dannon, 158
Brussels Sprouts, Glazed, 120

—C—

Cabbage
  Sweet and Sour, 136
  Turmeric, 119
Cake
  Breakfast, 21
  Orange Sponge, 170
Cannellini Roll-ups, 41
Carrots, Orange Glazed, 114
Cauliflower, Baked, 102
Cheese and Chicken Enchiladas, 133
Chicken
  and Pork Adobo, 131
  Arroz Con Pollo, 129
  Cutlets with Rosemary, 130
  Eat Like a Horse, 124
  Fajitas, 132
  Honey Mustard, 134
  Oven Baked "Fried", 126
  Piccata, 128
  Tandoori, 127
  Yakitori, 125

Chili
  Blanco, 139
  Vegetarian, 152
Chocolate Cupcakes with Mint Glaze, 169
Chocolate Mint Meltaways, 164
Chutney,
  Apricot, 51
  No-Cook, 50
Clams, Grilled, 39
Coconut Kisses, 160
Cole Slaw, Ruddy Good, 57
Cookies, Pepper, 155
Corn Chips, Oven-crisped, 32
Corn Pancakes, 116
Corn Pudding, 103
Corn Relish, 53
Corn, Creamed with Zucchini, 121
Cous Cous Primavera with Currants, 104
Crostini, Herbed, 40

—D—

Devil's Sauce, 47
Dressing
  Adults Only, 70
  Blue Cheese, 71
  Buttermilk, 66
  Caesar, 72
  Honey (for fruit salad), 68
  Honey Herb, 65
  Ranch, 67

—E—

Eggplant Dip, 42
Eggs
  Sardou, 24
  southwestern, 22

—F—

Fettuccine
    Alfredo with Crab, 90
    Spinach with Lemon
    Ricotta Sauce, 89
Fish, Baked, 145
Flan, Low Fat, 157
Floating Island, Librada's, 156
Frittata, 25

—G—

Game Hens, Glazed, 135
Garbanzos, Nutty Beans, 37
Garlic, Roasted, 30
Gnocchi with Pork and Carrots, 96
Granola, 18
Green Beans
    Hungarian, 101
    Sesame Seed, 100
Guacamole, Mock Guac, 33

—J—

Jalapeño Dip, 35
Jalapeño Jelly, 54

—L—

Lasagna, Gorgonzola, 86
Lemon Crunch, Frozen, 168

—M—

Money Bags, 137
Mushrooms, Roquefort, 29

—O—

Oatmeal, microwave, 16
Oranges in Wine, 159
Orzo with Herbs, 108

—P—

Pasta Primavera, 95
Pasta Salad
    Salmon, 92
    Tuna, 88
Pasta Sauce, Crock Pot, 87
Pea Pods, Stir-fried, 122
Peaches, Pretty, 167
Pears, Poached, 165
Pickles, Bread and Butter, 48
Pie Crust, No Fat, 166
Pie, Pavlova, 154
Pinto Beans, Frijomole, 34
Pintos Rancheros, 111
Pizza Sauce, Quick, 151
Pizza, 150
Popcorn, Ragin' Cajun, 36
Popovers, 19
Pork
    Skillet and Cabbage, 149
    Sweet and Sour, 148
Potato Onion Pie, 115
Potato Salad, Simply Scrumptious Creamy, 105
Potatoes
    Rosemary Roasted in Foil, 117
    Twice-Baked, 106

—R—

Raisin Sauce, Quick, 49
Ratatouille, Easy, 112
Rice
    Baked Yellow, 113
    Spanish, 109
Rigatoni with Mushroom Sauce, 94

—S—

Salad
    Black Bean, 56

Cherry Tomato, 61
Composed Tomato and
  Mozzarella, 63
Cucumber, 58
Raita, 62
Sauerkraut, 60
Shredded Carrot, 59
Salmon Croquettes, 144
Salsa, Mango, 44
  Pineapple, 52
  Verde, 45
Sauerbrauten, Same Day, 147
Shells Florentine, 97
Shrimp Étouffée, 143
Shrimp Fiesta, 142
Shrimp-Cucumber Dip, 38
Sloppy Jalopies, 138
Soup
  Black Bean with Shrimp, 80
  Escarole, 75
  Greek Lemon, 83
  Laurie Colwin's Curried
    Broccoli, 82
  Lentil & Brown Rice, 84
  Librada's Cloud, 74
  Macaroni, Bean and
    Spinach, 78
  One-Two-Three, 76
  Oriental Chicken, 77
  Pepper Cream, 79
  Velvet Summer Squash, 81
Spinach Soufflé, The World's
  Easiest, 110
Spinach with Chopped Egg, 121
Sweet Potato Pie, 118

—T—

Tapenade, 31
Tomatoes
  and Zucchini, Stewed, 121
  Stuffed Cherry, 28
Tubetti in Ricotta Pepper
  Sauce, 98
Tuna Creole with Angel Hair
  Pasta, 91
Turkey
  and Rice Green Pepper
    Boats, 140
  Picadillo, 141
  Tetrazzini, 93

—V—

Vinaigrette, Orange, 69

—Y—

Yellow Squash in Dill, 122
Yogurt and Fruit, 20

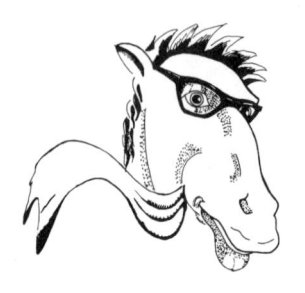

Here's an easy way to get more copies of Eat Like a Horse. Just fill out the information below.

Please send me ___ additional copies of EAT LIKE A HORSE AND LOSE WEIGHT at $11.95 per book. Add $3.00 per book and $1.00 for each additional book. Illinois residents add 7.75% sales tax.

Note: 10% discount for purchases of 5-9 books. 15% discount for purchases of 10 or more books with return of this card. Resellers please call for wholesale discount information.

Name: _____

Address (no P.O. Box): _____

City: _____ State: _____ Zip: _____

Telephone _____

_____ Check or money order enclosed.

Airplane Books, P.O. Box 111, Glenview, IL 60025 (708) 604-0602